Dosage Calculations Manual

Third Edition

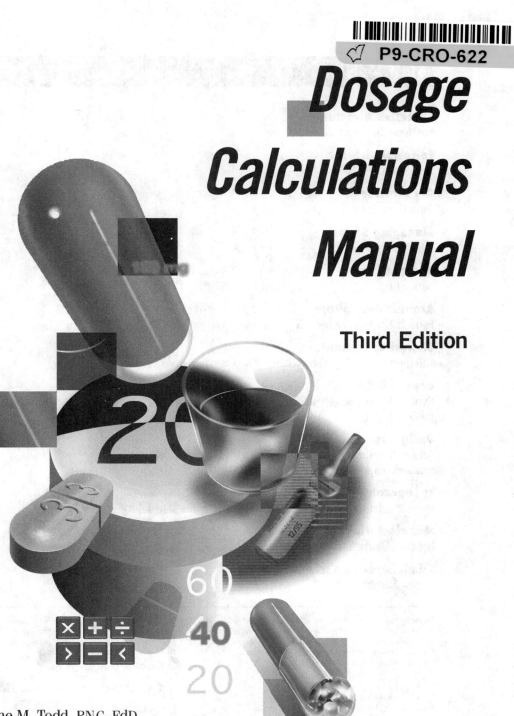

Catherine M. Todd, RN,C, EdD
Assistant Professor, Villanova University
College of Nursing, Villanova, Pennsylvania

Belle Erickson, RN,C, PhD
Assistant Professor, Villanova University
College of Nursing, Villanova, Pennsylvania

SPRINGHOUSE CORPORATION
SPRINGHOUSE, PENNSYLVANIA

Staff

Executive Director
Matthew Cahill

Editorial Director
June Norris

Art Director
John Hubbard

Managing Editor
David Moreau

Senior Editor
Nancy Priff

Acquisitions Editors
Patricia Kardish Fischer, RN, BSN; Louise Quinn

Clinical Consultants
Maryann Foley, RN, BSN; Collette Bishop Hendler, RN, CCRN

Copy Editors
Cynthia C. Breuninger (manager), Christine Cunniffe, Mary Teresa Durkin, Brenna Mayer, Patricia E. Polgar

Designers
Arlene Putterman (associate art director), Lorraine Lostracco, Susan Hopkins Rodzewich, Jeff Sklarow

Typography
Diane Paluba (manager), Joyce Rossi Biletz, Phyllis Marron, Valerie Rosenberger

Manufacturing
Deborah Meiris (director), Pat Dorshaw (manager), Anna Brindisi, T.A. Landis

Administrative Assistant
Jeanne Napier

© 1997 by Springhouse Corporation, 1111 Bethlehem Pike, P.O. Box 908, Springhouse, PA 19477-0908. All rights reserved. Reproduction in whole or part by any means whatsoever without written permission of the publisher is prohibited by law.

Printed in the United States of America.

ℛ A member of the Reed Elsevier plc group

DCM3E-020599

Library of Congress Cataloging-in-Publication Data
Todd, Catherine M.
Dosage calculations manual/Catherine M. Todd, Belle Erickson. – 3rd ed.
p. cm.
Includes index.
1. Pharmaceutical arithmetic. I. Erickson, Belle. II. Title.
RS57.T63 1992
615'.14 – dc20   96-32692
ISBN 0-87434-845-5 (alk. paper)   CIP

Contents

◆ UNIT 2: Systems of Drug Measurement

Chapter 6: Metric System

Chapter 7: Other Measurement Systems

◆ UNIT 3: Drug Orders and Medication Records

Chapter 8: Drug Orders

Chapter 9: Medication Records

◆ UNIT 4: Calculating Oral, Topical, and Rectal Dosages

Chapter 10: Oral Drug Labels

Chapter 11: Oral Drug Dosage Calculation

Chapter 12: Topical and Rectal Medications

◆ UNIT 5: Calculating Parenteral Dosages

Chapter 13: Syringes and Needles

Chapter 14: Parenteral Drugs and Labels

Chapter 15: Reconstitution and Use of Parenteral Drugs

Chapter 16: Insulin Dosage Calculations

Chapter 17: I.V. Flow Rate Calculations

Acknowledgments

Reviewer
David L. Wolff
Associate Professor
Montgomery County Community College
Blue Bell, Pa.

We thank the following companies for permission to use their drug labels.

Allen & Hanburys
Division of Glaxo Wellcome Inc.
Ventolin®

Altana Inc.
Nitrol® Ointment
Astra® USA, Inc.
Aquasol A®
Meperidine HCl Injection, USP
Streptase®

Biocraft Laboratories, Inc.
Oxacillin Sodium for Oral Solution USP

Bristol-Myers Squibb Company
Corgard®
Nafcillin Sodium for Injection USP
Pronestyl®
Vepesid®

Burroughs Wellcome Co.
Lanoxin®
Septra® Grape Suspension
Zovirax®

Dupont/Merck
Coumadin®
Narcan®
Percocet®

Eli Lilly and Company
Ceclor®
Dobutrex® Solution
Humulin® 70/30
Humulin®N
Humulin®R
Nebcin®
Quinidine Gluconate Injection USP

E.R. Squibb & Sons, Inc.
Principen®

G & W Labs
Morphine Sulfate
Truphyline™

G.D. Searle & Company
Flagyl®
Norpace®

Glaxo Pharmaceuticals
Zantac®

Hoechst Marion Roussel, Inc.
DiaBeta®
Lasix®
Norpramin®

Janssen Pharmaceutical, Inc.
Sublimaze®

Knoll Pharmaceutical Company
Synthroid®

Merck & Co., Inc.
Pepcid®
Prinivil®
Vasotec®
Zocor®

Novo Nordisk
Novolin®L
Novolin®N
Novolin®R

Ortho/McNeil Pharmaceutical
Monistat-Derm®
Retin-A®
Spectazole®
Tylenol®

Roxane Laboratories, Inc.
Prednisone Oral Solution USP

Sandoz Pharmaceuticals Corporation
Mellaril®

SmithKline Beecham Pharmaceuticals
Augmentin®
Bactroban®
Compazine®

Warner-Lambert Company
Dilantin®
Pitocin®

Dosage Calculations Manual, Third Edition, provides the information you need to calculate dosages confidently and prepare medications exactly as ordered. Designed for easy use, this manual presents patient situations for each new type of calculation, providing a step-by-step approach to computing drug dosages. The information on each type of calculation progresses from simple to complex. For example, it moves from calculations that require one step to those that require two or more computations to determine a dosage.

Because practicing dosage calculations is the best way to fine-tune this skill, *Dosage Calculations Manual,* Third Edition, provides many opportunities to do so. Its pretest assesses your basic mathematical skills and aids in focusing your studies. Practice questions at the end of each section and review questions at the end of every chapter give you a chance to test your expanding skills. In addition to the hundreds of practice and review questions, a comprehensive test before the appendices helps reinforce knowledge and identify areas that need further practice.

This edition offers new and expanded content, including a more extensive review of mathematical skills, new chapters on performing critical care calculations and selecting appropriate syringes and needles, updated information on computerized medication records and drug administration equipment, expanded coverage of pediatric calculations, and more. It also provides new features, such as numerous drug labels, and golden rules that highlight vital information.

From cover to cover, *Dosage Calculations Manual,* Third Edition, puts all the information you need at your fingertips. Unit 1, Review of Mathematics, begins with a pretest that assesses your ability to solve basic mathematical problems. Next it presents the use of fractions, decimals, percentages, ratios, and proportions. Then it shows how to set up and solve equations to find the value of X.

In Unit 2, Systems of Drug Measurement, the metric system is highlighted as the major system of drug weights and volume measures. Then the unit describes the apothecaries', household, avoirdupois, unit, and milliequivalent systems. It also explains how to convert measurements within and among these systems.

Unit 3, Drug Orders and Medication Records, explores drug orders, describing how to read them and deal with unclear orders. The unit then discusses medication record systems, highlighting accurate documentation, quality assurance, and error prevention and reporting.

Unit 4, Calculating Oral, Topical, and Rectal Dosages, demonstrates how to read drug labels. It also applies the mathematical skills presented in Unit 1 to dosage calculations involving tablets, capsules, oral solutions, and topical and rectal drugs.

After introducing the syringes and needles used for drug administration, Unit 5, Calculating Parenteral Dosages, describes how to read parenteral solution labels and how to measure, reconstitute, and use parenteral drugs. The unit continues with insulin therapy, featuring the special equipment, orders, and calculations required. Next, it addresses I.V. fluid and medication administration, presenting I.V. flow rate, drip rate, and infusion-time calculations as well as information about equipment— from basic administration sets to patient-controlled analgesia infusion pumps. The unit concludes with specialized calculations related to I.V. medications, such as heparin, aminophylline, electrolytes, and nutrients.

Unit 6, Special Dosage Calculations, describes the computations needed to calculate pediatric dosages (based on the child's body weight and body surface area, among other methods) and pediatric fluid needs. It also reviews significant factors to consider for patients of all ages who require individualized dosages, such as obstetric and critical care patients.

The main text concludes with a 148-item comprehensive test to evaluate your mastery of all information presented. For ready reference, the book includes six useful appendices, updated references, and a comprehensive index.

Dosage Calculations Manual, Third Edition, is the ideal resource for anyone who prepares and administers drugs. Professional nurses can use the manual when an unfamiliar calculation is required, a computation must be verified, or a refresher is needed. Nursing students can use the manual to learn and practice calculation skills needed for safe and accurate drug administration.

UNIT 1

◆

Review of Mathematics

Accurately performing mathematical calculations is essential to nurses, especially when administering medications and intravenous fluids. Although many facilities use the unit-dose drug distribution system, which reduces the time spent calculating dosages, you must know how to perform accurate calculations to confirm that a patient receives correct dosages. You also need sharp mathematical skills to calculate dosages of medications that are available only in fixed concentrations or strengths. Therefore, you must be able to use fractions, decimals, percentages, ratios, and proportions properly and to set up equations to solve for the value of X. Once the value of X is calculated, you can determine the appropriate dosage or flow rate for administering the medication or fluid to the patient.

To prepare you for these tasks, Unit 1 reviews the mathematical calculations that form the foundation of virtually all of the medication calculations you'll need in nursing. The unit covers fractions, decimals, percentages, and ratios and fractions in proportions. Then using this information, it illustrates how to solve problems to find the value of X.

Before you read the rest of this unit, take the Pretest to assess your ability to perform basic mathematical calculations. Then, use the information in the unit to review and strengthen your abilities. As you move through each chapter, test yourself with practice problems, which appear after each topic, and with review problems, which appear at the end of each chapter. To check your calculations, simply turn to the answers, which conclude each chapter.

Pretest

This pretest will help assess your knowledge of basic mathematical concepts and the ability to solve common arithmetic problems. To check your answers, see pages 4 to 6.

1. In the fraction ²/₇, which number is the numerator and which is the denominator?
2. Of the fractions ½, ⁶/₇, and ⁷/₆, which is the improper fraction?
3. Reduce the following fractions to their lowest terms.
   a) ⁴/₆
   b) ²⁵/₁₀₀
   c) ⁶/₁₈
4. Of the numbers 2, 5, and 9, which one is not a prime factor?
5. For the fractions ⅕, ⅙, and ⅛, what is the lowest common denominator?

6. Add the following sets of fractions.

   a) ⅔ + ⅙ + ⅖

   b) ⅒ + ¹⁄₁₅ + ⅙

   c) ⅐ + ⅛ + ²⁄₉

7. Subtract the following fractions.

   a) ⅞ − ¾

   b) ⅔ − ¼

   c) ⅙ − ⅛

8. Multiply the following fractions.

   a) ²⁄₇ × ⁸⁄₉

   b) 1½ × ⅞

   c) 3¼ × 5⅛

9. Simplify the following complex fractions.

   a) $\dfrac{⁶⁄₇}{⅞}$

   b) $\dfrac{⅔}{³⁄₇}$

   c) $\dfrac{⅚}{⅓}$

10. Divide the following fractions.

   a) 1½ ÷ ⅔

   b) ⅞ ÷ ⅘

   c) ⁴⁄₇ ÷ ⅚

11. For each of the following decimal fractions, what number is in the hundredths place?

   a) 3.124

   b) 0.1057

   c) 12.879

12. Round off the following decimal fractions to the nearest tenth.

   a) 8.245

   b) 10.2367

   c) 0.252

13. Add the following decimal fractions.

   a) 0.234 + 1.1

   b) 7.3 + 4.578 + 9.07

   c) 0.456 + 0.06 + 8.97

14. Subtract the following decimal fractions.

   a) 10.005 − 0.05

   b) 0.75 − 0.025

   c) 1.5 − 0.005

15. Multiply the following decimal fractions.

    a) 4.5×0.025

    b) 2.1×10.003

    c) 9.1×0.2

16. Convert the following decimal fractions to common fractions.

    a) 0.25

    b) 0.64

    c) 1.85

17. Convert the following percentages to decimal fractions.

    a) 85%

    b) 67%

18. Convert the following percentages to common fractions.

    a) 40%

    b) 75%

19. Convert the following common fractions to percentages.

    a) $\frac{3}{8}$

    b) $\frac{2}{3}$

    c) $\frac{9}{10}$

20. Convert the following decimal fractions to percentages.

    a) 0.257

    b) 0.86

    c) 0.054

21. What is 35% of 100?

22. 150 is what percent of 1,000?

23. Express the following ratios as fractions in proportions.

    a) $2:5::4:10$

    b) $1:3::4:12$

    c) $6:9::2:3$

24. Express the following fractions as ratios in proportions.

    a) $\frac{1}{3} = \frac{3}{9}$

    b) $\frac{5}{1} = \frac{10}{2}$

    c) $\frac{6}{7} = \frac{30}{35}$

25. Solve for X in the following proportions, which are expressed using fractions.

    a) $\dfrac{1}{2} = \dfrac{X}{8}$

    b) $\dfrac{23}{59} = \dfrac{3}{X}$

    c) $\dfrac{9}{3} = \dfrac{X}{27}$

26. Solve for X in the following proportions, which are expressed using ratios.

    a) $3:10 = 12:X$

    b) $5: 6 = 7:X$

    c) $0.5:10 = 5:X$

Answers to Pretest

1. 2 is the numerator, 7 is the denominator.

2. $7/6$ is the improper fraction.

3. a) $2/3$

    b) $1/4$

    c) $1/3$

4. 9 is not a prime factor, because it is divisible by 3.

5. 120 is the lowest common denominator:
$1/5 = 24/120, 1/6 = 20/120, 1/8 = 15/120$

6. a) $2/3 + 1/6 + 2/5 = 20/30 + 5/30 + 12/30 = 37/30 = 1 7/30$

    b) $1/10 + 1/15 + 1/6 = 3/30 + 2/30 + 5/30 = 10/30 = 1/3$

    c) $1/7 + 1/8 + 2/9 = 72/504 + 63/504 + 112/504 = 247/504$

7. a) $7/8 - 3/4 = 7/8 - 6/8 = 1/8$

    b) $2/3 - 1/4 = 8/12 - 3/12 = 5/12$

    c) $1/6 - 1/8 = 4/24 - 3/24 = 1/24$

8. a) $2/7 \times 8/9 = 16/63$

    b) $1 1/2 \times 7/8 = 3/2 \times 7/8 = 21/16 = 1 5/16$

    c) $3 1/4 \times 5 1/8 = 13/4 \times 41/8 = 533/32 = 16 21/32$

9. a) $6/7 \times 8/7 = 48/49$

    b) $2/3 \times 7/3 = 14/9 = 1 5/9$

    c) $5/6 \times 3/1 = 15/6 = 2 3/6 = 2 1/2$

10. a) $1 1/2 \div 2/3 = 3/2 \times 3/2 = 9/4 = 2 1/4$

    b) $7/8 \div 4/5 = 7/8 \times 5/4 = 35/32 = 1 3/32$

    c) $4/7 \div 5/6 = 4/7 \times 6/5 = 24/35$

11. a) 2

    b) 0

    c) 7

12. a) 8.2

    b) 10.2

    c) 0.3

13. a)
$$\begin{array}{r} 0.234 \\ +\ 1.100 \\ \hline 1.334 \end{array}$$

b)
$$\begin{array}{r} 7.300 \\ 4.578 \\ +\ 9.070 \\ \hline 20.948 \end{array}$$

c)
$$\begin{array}{r} 0.456 \\ 0.060 \\ +\ 8.970 \\ \hline 9.486 \end{array}$$

14. a)
$$\begin{array}{r} 10.005 \\ -\ 0.050 \\ \hline 9.955 \end{array}$$

b)
$$\begin{array}{r} 0.750 \\ -\ 0.025 \\ \hline 0.725 \end{array}$$

c)
$$\begin{array}{r} 1.500 \\ -\ 0.005 \\ \hline 1.495 \end{array}$$

15. a)
$$\begin{array}{r} 0.025 \\ \times\ 4.5 \\ \hline 0.1125 \end{array}$$

b)
$$\begin{array}{r} 10.003 \\ \times\ 2.1 \\ \hline 21.0063 \end{array}$$

c)
$$\begin{array}{r} 9.1 \\ \times\ 0.2 \\ \hline 1.82 \end{array}$$

16. a) $0.25 = {}^{25}\!/_{100} = {}^{1}\!/_{4}$

b) $0.64 = {}^{64}\!/_{100} = {}^{16}\!/_{25}$

c) $1.85 = 1{}^{85}\!/_{100} = 1{}^{17}\!/_{20}$

17. a) $85 \times 0.01 = 0.85$
(or remove the percent sign and move the decimal point two places to the left)

b) $67 \times 0.01 = 0.67$
(or remove the percent sign and move the decimal point two places to the left)

18. a) $40\% = 0.40 = {}^{40}\!/_{100} = {}^{2}\!/_{5}$

b) $75\% = 0.75 = {}^{75}\!/_{100} = {}^{3}\!/_{4}$

19. a) ${}^{3}\!/_{8} = 0.375 = 37.5\%$ (or 38%, if rounded)

b) ${}^{2}\!/_{3} = 0.666 = 66.6\%$ (or 67%, if rounded)

c) ${}^{9}\!/_{10} = 0.90 = 90\%$

20. a) $0.257 = 25.7\%$ (or move the decimal point two places to the right and add the percent sign)

b) $0.86 = 86\%$ (or move the decimal point two places to the right and add the percent sign)

c) $0.054 = 5.4\%$ (or move the decimal point two places to the right and add the percent sign)

21. $100 \times 0.35 = 35$

22. $150 \div 1,000 = 0.15 = 15\%$

23. a) $\frac{2}{5} = \frac{4}{10}$

b) $\frac{1}{3} = \frac{4}{12}$

c) $\frac{6}{9} = \frac{2}{3}$

24. a) $1:3 = 3:9$

b) $5:1 = 10:2$

c) $6:7 = 30:35$

25. a) $\dfrac{1}{2} = \dfrac{X}{8}$

$1 \times 8 = 2 \times X$

$\dfrac{8}{2} = X$

$4 = X$

b) $\dfrac{23}{59} = \dfrac{3}{X}$

$23 \times X = 59 \times 3$

$23X = 177$

$X = \dfrac{177}{23}$

$X = 7.69$ (or 7.7, if rounded)

c) $\dfrac{9}{3} = \dfrac{X}{27}$

$9 \times 27 = 3 \times X$

$243 = 3X$

$\dfrac{243}{3} = X$

$81 = X$

26. a) $3:10 = 12:X$

$3X = 120$

$X = 40$

b) $5:6 = 7:X$

$5X = 42$

$X = 8\frac{2}{5}$

c) $0.5:10 = 5:X$

$0.5X = 50$

$X = 100$

Chapter

1

◆

Fractions

A fraction represents a mathematical expression for parts of a whole. It appears as one number over another separated by a short line.

The bottom number, or *denominator,* represents the total number of equal parts in the whole. The larger the denominator, the greater the number of equal parts. For example, in the fraction ⅔, the denominator 3 indicates that the whole has been divided into three equal parts. In the fraction ⁵⁄₁₆, the denominator 16 indicates that the whole has been divided into 16 equal parts. Thus, as the denominator becomes larger, the size of the parts becomes smaller.

The top number, or *numerator,* signifies the number of parts of the whole being considered. For example, in the fraction ⅔, only 2 of the 3 equal parts are being considered. In the fraction ⁵⁄₁₆, only 5 of the 16 equal parts are being considered. (See *Parts of a whole,* page 8, for an illustration of this concept.)

In a *common fraction,* such as ⅚, the numerator and denominator are both whole numbers. In a *complex fraction,* the numerator and denominator are fractions themselves, such as:

$$\frac{\frac{1}{4}}{\frac{5}{16}}$$

A *proper fraction* describes any fraction with a numerator smaller than the denominator, such as ⅜. The term *improper fraction* refers to any fraction with a numerator larger than the denominator, such as ⁹⁄₈ or ¹²⁄₅. In such a fraction, more than one whole is being considered. For convenience, improper fractions are usually expressed as *mixed numbers,* or numbers that consist of a whole number and a fraction; therefore, ⁹⁄₈ becomes 1⅛ and ¹²⁄₅ becomes 2⅖.

Three techniques are frequently used with fractions: converting between mixed numbers and improper fractions, reducing fractions to the lowest terms, and finding the lowest common denominator.

Converting between mixed numbers and improper fractions

To convert mixed numbers to improper fractions, multiply the denominator by the whole number and add the numerator. For example, to convert the mixed number 7⅝ to an improper fraction, multiply the denominator 8 by the whole number 7, for a total of 56. Then add 56 to the numerator 5, for a new numerator of 61. Leaving the denominator the same, the improper fraction is ⁶¹⁄₈. In another example, to convert 8⅘ to an improper fraction, multiply the denominator 5 by the whole number 8, for a total of 40. Then add 40 to the numerator 4, for a new numerator of 44. Leaving the denominator the same, the improper fraction is ⁴⁴⁄₅.

Parts of a whole

In any fraction, the numerator (top number) and denominator (bottom number) tell something about the parts of a whole. The denominator describes the total number of equal parts in the whole; the numerator describes the number of parts being considered, as illustrated below.

TWO-THIRDS (⅔)

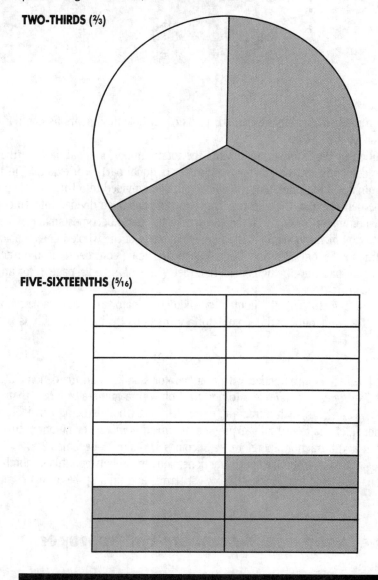

FIVE-SIXTEENTHS (⁵⁄₁₆)

To convert an improper fraction to a mixed number, reverse this process. In the first example, divide the numerator 61 by the denominator 8 to obtain 7 with a remainder of ⅝, or 7⅝; in the second example, divide the numerator 44 by the denominator 5 to obtain 8 with a remainder of ⅘, or 8⅘.

PRACTICE PROBLEMS

Converting between mixed numbers and improper fractions

Calculate the solutions to the following questions about fractions. To check your answers, see page 16.

1. Convert the following mixed numbers to improper fractions.
   a) 4⅔
   b) 12³⁄₇
   c) 5⅚
   d) 9½

2. Convert the following improper fractions to mixed numbers.
   a) ⁸⁄₅
   b) ¹⁵⁄₁₁
   c) ²¹⁄₆

Reducing fractions to the lowest terms

Usually, fractions should be reduced to their lowest terms. To simplify a fraction, determine the largest common divisor (a number into which another number can be divided evenly) of the numerator and the denominator and divide them both by that number. In the fraction ⁴⁄₆, for example, 2 is the largest divisor that 4 and 6 have in common. Dividing the numerator and denominator by 2 reduces the fraction to its lowest terms, ⅔.

◆ **PRACTICE PROBLEMS**

Reducing fractions to the lowest terms

Reduce the following fractions to their lowest terms. To check your answers, see page 16.

1. ⁷⁄₁₄
2. ¹⁸⁄₂₄
3. ²⁄₁₀
4. ⁸⁄₄₈

Finding the lowest common denominator

Another useful tool for handling fractions is the lowest common denominator (LCD). This is the smallest number that is a multiple of the known denominators (the least common multiple, or LCM). The easiest method for finding a common denominator is to multiply all the denominators. For example, to find the common denominator for ½ and ⅙, multiply 2 by 6 (2 × 6 = 12). However, this may not give you the *lowest* common denominator, which will be easier to work with than a larger common denominator. To find the LCD, list each denominator and its prime factors (numbers that are evenly divisible by only 1 and themselves, such as 2, 3, 5, and 7).

Use prime factoring to find the LCD for ¹⁄₁₂, ¼, and ⅕, where a multiplied common denominator would be 240 (12 × 4 × 5).

◆ Make a horizontal list of the denominators. Then, divide these by the prime factors for each, starting with the smallest prime factor that divides into one of the denominators—in this case, 2. Bring down to the next line any numbers that are not evenly divisible by a prime factor. Repeat this process until the numbers in the bottom row can be divided no further.

Prime Factors	Denominators		
	12	4	5
2	6	2	5
2	3	1	5

◆ Multiply all the prime factors in the left column by each number in the bottom row.

$$2 \times 2 \times 3 \times 1 \times 5 = 60.$$

The LCD for this set of fractions is 60.

Use prime factoring to find the LCD for ⅛, ½, and ⅓, where a multiplied common denominator is 48 (8 × 2 × 3).

◆ Make a horizontal list of denominators and divide these by the prime factors, as above.

Prime Factors	Denominators		
	8	2	3
2	4	1	3
2	2	1	3

◆ Multiply all the prime factors in the left column by each number in the bottom row.

$$2 \times 2 \times 2 \times 1 \times 3 = 24$$

The LCD for this set of fractions is 24.

Another way to use prime factoring to find the LCD is to list the denominators vertically. Then factor each number, lining up the factors in columns. Bring down the factors from each column and multiply them to find the LCD. For the fractions ¹⁄₁₂, ¼, and ⅕, you can use this method to find the LCD as shown below.

$$\begin{array}{l} \text{Denominators} \quad \text{Prime Factors} \\ 12 = 2 \times 2 \times 3 \\ 4 = 2 \times 2 \\ 5 = \underline{\qquad\qquad 1 \times 5} \\ 2 \times 2 \times 3 \times 1 \times 5 = 60 \end{array}$$

The LCD is 60.

For the fractions ⅛, ½, and ⅓, use the same method to find the LCD.

$$\begin{array}{l} \text{Denominators} \quad \text{Prime Factors} \\ 8 = 2 \times 2 \times 2 \\ 2 = 2 \times 1 \\ 3 = \underline{\qquad\qquad 1 \times 3} \\ 2 \times 2 \times 2 \times 1 \times 3 = 24 \end{array}$$

The LCD is 24.

Convert $\frac{1}{12}$, $\frac{1}{4}$, and $\frac{1}{5}$ to fractions with the LCD. Multiply each by 1 in the form of a fraction (in which the numerator and denominator are the same number) that will yield the LCD — in this case, 60.

$$\frac{1}{12} \times \frac{5}{5} = \frac{5}{60}$$
$$\frac{1}{4} \times \frac{15}{15} = \frac{15}{60}$$
$$\frac{1}{5} \times \frac{12}{12} = \frac{12}{60}$$

In the second example, convert $\frac{1}{8}$, $\frac{1}{2}$, and $\frac{1}{3}$ to fractions with the LCD. In this case, the LCD is 24.

$$\frac{1}{8} \times \frac{3}{3} = \frac{3}{24}$$
$$\frac{1}{2} \times \frac{12}{12} = \frac{12}{24}$$
$$\frac{1}{3} \times \frac{8}{8} = \frac{8}{24}$$

Another way to convert the fractions is to divide each denominator into the LCD — in this case, 60. Then multiply the numerator by the number obtained to determine the new numerator for the fraction with a denominator of 60.

$$\frac{1}{12} = 12\overline{)60} \quad 5 \times 1 = \frac{5}{60}$$

$$\frac{1}{4} = 4\overline{)60} \quad 15 \times 1 = \frac{15}{60}$$

$$\frac{1}{5} = 5\overline{)60} \quad 12 \times 1 = \frac{12}{60}$$

Or, as in the second example,

$$\frac{1}{8} = 8\overline{)24} \quad 3 \times 1 = \frac{3}{24}$$

$$\frac{1}{2} = 2\overline{)24} \quad 12 \times 1 = \frac{12}{24}$$

$$\frac{1}{3} = 3\overline{)24} \quad 8 \times 1 = \frac{8}{24}$$

(See "Multiplying fractions" for further details.)

Finding the LCD in a group of fractions allows you to compare the fractions. The LCD, for example, would allow you to compare the strengths of sublingual nitroglycerin tablets, which are available in $\frac{1}{100}$-, $\frac{1}{150}$-, and $\frac{1}{200}$-grain strengths.

Find the LCD for $\frac{1}{100}$, $\frac{1}{150}$, and $\frac{1}{200}$ to compare these strengths.

◆ Begin by making a vertical list of the denominators and factoring each number. Bring down the factors in each column; then multiply them to find the LCD.

$$100 = 2 \times 2 \times 5 \times 5$$
$$150 = 2 \times 5 \times 5 \times 3$$
$$200 = \underline{2 \times 2 \times 2 \times 5 \times 5}$$
$$2 \times 2 \times 2 \times 5 \times 5 \times 3 = 600$$

The LCD is 600.

◆ Convert all of the fractions to new fractions with the LCD—in this case, 600. To do this, multiply by 1 in the form of a fraction (such as ⁶⁄₆, ⁴⁄₄, or ³⁄₃), or divide each denominator into 600 and then multiply its numerator by the number obtained, as shown below.

$$100\overline{\smash{\big)}600} \qquad 6 \times 1 = {}^{6}\!/_{600}$$

$$150\overline{\smash{\big)}600} \qquad 4 \times 1 = {}^{4}\!/_{600}$$

$$200\overline{\smash{\big)}600} \qquad 3 \times 1 = {}^{3}\!/_{600}$$

The ¹⁄₁₀₀-grain nitroglycerin tablet would offer the largest dose (⁶⁄₆₀₀).

When comparing fractions with common denominators, remember that the fraction with the largest numerator represents the largest number. This is true only when the denominators are the same. So, to compare common fractions, convert them to fractions with common denominators. To compare such complex fractions as

$$\frac{{}^{1}\!/_{4}}{{}^{5}\!/_{6}} \text{ and } \frac{{}^{2}\!/_{3}}{{}^{4}\!/_{5}}$$

Simplify them by treating the line between each complex fraction's numerator and denominator as a division sign. (See "Dividing fractions" for further information.)

Finding the LCD also allows you to add and subtract fractions. Reducing fractions to the lowest terms and converting improper fractions to mixed numbers allows you to present the answers to addition, subtraction, multiplication, and division problems in a useful way. Whenever you perform these functions, always reduce the final answer to its lowest terms and, if it is an improper fraction, convert it to a mixed number.

◆ PRACTICE PROBLEMS

Finding the lowest common denominator

Find the LCD for the following fractions. To check your answers, see page 17.

1. ¹⁄₃, ¹⁄₄, ¹⁄₆

2. ³⁄₈, ⁵⁄₆

3. ²⁄₃, ⁴⁄₉, ¹⁄₆

4. ¹⁄₈, ¹⁄₅, ¹⁄₄

Adding fractions

To add fractions, convert them to fractions with common denominators. Using the method described above, multiply by 1 in the form of a fraction to convert them to fractions with the LCD.

Add ½ and ⅓.

◆ Multiply each by 1 in the form of a fraction to yield fractions with the LCD 6.

$${}^{1}\!/_{2} \times {}^{3}\!/_{3} = {}^{3}\!/_{6}$$

$${}^{1}\!/_{3} \times {}^{2}\!/_{2} = {}^{2}\!/_{6}$$

◆ Now that the fractions have common denominators, add them by adding the new numerators and placing the result over the common denominator. Then reduce the fractions, if possible.

$${}^{3}\!/_{6} + {}^{2}\!/_{6} = {}^{5}\!/_{6}$$

Add $1/4$ and $1/5$.

- Multiply each by 1 in the form of a fraction to yield factors with the LCD 20.

$$1/4 \times 5/5 = 5/20$$
$$1/5 \times 4/4 = 4/20$$

- Add the new numerators and place the result over the common denominator. Then reduce, if possible.

$$5/20 + 4/20 = 9/20$$

◆ PRACTICE PROBLEMS

Adding fractions

Add the following fractions. To check your answers, see page 17.

1. $1/10 + 1/5 + 1/4$
2. $3/5 + 2/3$
3. $5/36 + 1/6 + 1/4$
4. $1\,2/3 + 7\,7/12 + 2\,3/4$

Subtracting fractions

As in addition, subtraction of fractions requires converting them to fractions with common denominators.

Subtract $3/5$ from $7/8$.

- First change them to fractions with the LCD – in this case, 40. Multiply each fraction by the number 1 in the form of a fraction to yield a denominator of 40.

$$7/8 \times 5/5 = 35/40$$
$$3/5 \times 8/8 = 24/40$$

- Now that the fractions have common denominators, subtract them by subtracting the numerators and placing the result over the common denominator. Then reduce, if possible.

$$35/40 - 24/40 = 11/40$$

Subtract $2/3$ from $4/5$.

- Multiply each fraction by the number 1 in the form of a fraction to yield a denominator of 15.

$$4/5 \times 3/3 = 12/15$$
$$2/3 \times 5/5 = 10/15$$

- Then subtract the numerators and place the result over the common denominator. Then reduce, if possible.

$$12/15 - 10/15 = 2/15$$

◆ PRACTICE PROBLEMS

Subtracting fractions

Subtract the following fractions. To check your answers, see page 17.

1. $2/3 - 1/4$
2. $5/12 - 1/6$
3. $1\,1/2 - 3/8$
4. $4/5 - 2/3$

Multiplying fractions

You can multiply or divide fractions without converting to common denominators. To multiply fractions, multiply the numerators and denominators in turn.

Multiply ¼ by ⅞.
* Multiply the numerators ($1 \times 7 = 7$) for a new numerator of 7. Then multiply the denominators ($4 \times 8 = 32$) for a new denominator of 32.

$$\tfrac{1}{4} \times \tfrac{7}{8} = \frac{1 \times 7}{4 \times 8} = \tfrac{7}{32}$$

Multiply ⅔ × 3/7.
* Multiply the numerators ($2 \times 3 = 6$) for a new numerator of 6; then multiply the denominators ($3 \times 7 = 21$) for a new denominator of 21.

$$\tfrac{2}{3} \times \tfrac{3}{7} = \frac{2 \times 3}{3 \times 7} = \tfrac{6}{21}$$

To multiply fractions by whole numbers, convert the whole number to a fraction.

Multiply ⅜ by 2.
* First convert 2 to the fraction 2/1. Then multiply as described above. The complete calculation should look like this, with the answer reduced to its lowest terms:

$$\tfrac{3}{8} \times 2 = \frac{3}{8} \times \frac{2}{1} = \frac{3 \times 2}{8 \times 1} = \frac{6}{8} = \tfrac{3}{4}$$

Multiply 2/7 by 3, using the same method.

$$\tfrac{2}{7} \times 3 = \frac{2}{7} \times \frac{3}{1} = \frac{2 \times 3}{7 \times 1} = \tfrac{6}{7}$$

◆ **PRACTICE PROBLEMS**

Multiplying fractions

Multiply the following fractions. To check your answers, see page 17.

1. ⅖ × ⅚
2. 4/7 × ⅝
3. ⅓ × 4/11 × ½
4. 1½ × 2⅔ × ⅙

Dividing fractions

Division problems are usually written as two fractions separated by a division sign, such as ⅘ ÷ ⅔. In this problem, the first fraction (⅘) is the *dividend,* the number to be divided; the second one (⅔) is the *divisor.* To divide a fraction, multiply by the divisor's *reciprocal* (inverted fraction).

Divide ⅘ by ⅔.
* Multiply the dividend by the reciprocal of the divisor—in this case, 3/2. Then reduce the answer to its lowest terms.

$$\tfrac{4}{5} \div \tfrac{2}{3} = \frac{4}{5} \times \frac{3}{2} = \frac{4 \times 3}{5 \times 2} = \frac{12}{10} = 1 = 1\tfrac{1}{5}$$

Divide 5/6 by 1/3, using the same method.

$$5/6 \div 1/3 = \frac{5}{6} \times \frac{3}{1} = \frac{5 \times 3}{6 \times 1} = \frac{15}{6} = 2\,3/6 = 2\,1/2$$

To divide a fraction by a whole number, use the same principle. For easier handling, first convert the divisor to a fraction. Then invert the divisor to obtain its reciprocal and multiply.

Divide 2/3 by 4.

- First convert the whole number to a fraction (4/1). Then multiply the dividend by the reciprocal of the divisor—in this case, 1/4. Then reduce the answer to its lowest terms.

$$2/3 \div 4 = \frac{2}{3} \div \frac{4}{1} = \frac{2}{3} \times \frac{1}{4} = \frac{2 \times 1}{3 \times 4} = \frac{2}{12} = 1/6$$

Divide 4/5 by 3, using the same method.

$$4/5 \div 3 = \frac{4}{5} \div \frac{3}{1} = \frac{4}{5} \times \frac{1}{3} = \frac{4 \times 1}{5 \times 3} = 4/15$$

To divide complex fractions, follow the same rules. The calculation, for example, might look like this with the answer reduced to the lowest terms and converted to a mixed number:

$$\frac{1/4}{3/16} = \frac{1}{4} \div \frac{3}{16} = \frac{1}{4} \times \frac{16}{3} = \frac{1 \times 16}{4 \times 3} = \frac{16}{12} = 1\,4/12 = 1\,1/3$$

Here is another example:

$$\frac{4/7}{2/5} = \frac{4}{7} \div \frac{2}{5} = \frac{4}{7} \times \frac{5}{2} = \frac{4 \times 5}{7 \times 2} = \frac{20}{14} = 1\,6/14 = 1\,3/7$$

◆ PRACTICE PROBLEMS

Dividing fractions

Divide the following fractions. To check your answers, see page 17.

1. 5/7 ÷ 2/3
2. 6 3/5 ÷ 2 1/3
3. 1/4 ÷ 1/3
4. 8/2 ÷ 10/6

Review problems

Calculate the solutions to the following questions about fractions. To check your answers, see pages 17 and 18.

1. In the fraction 7/16, which number is the numerator and which is the denominator?
2. Of the fractions 2/3, 10/9, and 9/10, which is the improper fraction?
3. Reduce the following fractions to their lowest terms.
   a) 75/100
   b) 4/6
   c) 2/8
4. Of the numbers 7, 4, and 8, which one is a prime factor?
5. For the fractions 2/3, 5/6, and 3/8, what is the LCD?

6. Add the following sets of fractions.

   a) $\frac{9}{10} + \frac{2}{3} + \frac{1}{5}$

   b) $\frac{1}{4} + \frac{4}{7} + \frac{3}{8}$

   c) $\frac{5}{12} + \frac{2}{5} + \frac{7}{8}$

7. Subtract the following fractions.

   a) $\frac{5}{8} - \frac{1}{4}$

   b) $\frac{1}{3} - \frac{1}{4}$

   c) $\frac{7}{16} - \frac{3}{8}$

8. Multiply the following fractions.

   a) $9\frac{1}{4} \times \frac{1}{8}$

   b) $\frac{2}{9} \times \frac{4}{7}$

   c) $6\frac{1}{2} \times 4\frac{3}{8}$

9. Simplify the following complex fractions.

   a) $\dfrac{\frac{2}{3}}{\frac{7}{8}}$

   b) $\dfrac{\frac{5}{7}}{\frac{3}{4}}$

   c) $\dfrac{\frac{5}{3}}{\frac{7}{8}}$

10. Divide the following fractions.

    a) $\frac{4}{5} \div \frac{2}{3}$

    b) $\frac{7}{8} \div 1\frac{1}{2}$

    c) $\frac{5}{6} \div \frac{4}{7}$

Answers to practice problems

◆ Converting between mixed numbers and improper fractions

1. a) $\frac{14}{3}$

   b) $\frac{87}{7}$

   c) $\frac{35}{6}$

   d) $\frac{19}{2}$

2. a) $1\frac{3}{5}$

   b) $1\frac{4}{11}$

   c) $3\frac{3}{6} = 3\frac{1}{2}$

◆ Reducing fractions to lowest terms

1. $\frac{7}{14} = \frac{1}{2}$

2. $\frac{18}{24} = \frac{3}{4}$

3. $\frac{2}{10} = \frac{1}{5}$

4. $\frac{8}{48} = \frac{1}{6}$

♦ *Finding the lowest common denominator*

1. 12

2. 24

3. 18

4. 40

♦ *Adding fractions*

1. $^{11}/_{20}$

2. $^{19}/_{15} = 1^4/_{15}$

3. $^{20}/_{36} = ^5/_9$

4. $^{144}/_{12} = 12$

♦ *Subtracting fractions*

1. $^5/_{12}$

2. $^3/_{12} = ^1/_4$

3. $^9/_8 = 1^1/_8$

4. $^2/_{15}$

♦ *Multiplying fractions*

1. $^{10}/_{30} = ^1/_3$

2. $^{20}/_{56} = ^5/_{14}$

3. $^4/_{66} = ^2/_{33}$

4. $^{24}/_{36} = ^2/_3$

♦ *Dividing fractions*

1. $^{15}/_{14} = 1^1/_{14}$

2. $^{99}/_{35} = 2^{29}/_{35}$

3. $^3/_4$

4. $^{48}/_{20} = 2^2/_5$

Answers to review problems

1. 7 is the numerator; 16 is the denominator.

2. $^{10}/_9$ is the improper fraction.

3. a) $^3/_4$

   b) $^2/_3$

   c) $^1/_4$

4. 7 is a prime factor.

5. 24 is the LCD.

6. a) $^{53}/_{30} = 1^{23}/_{30}$

   b) $^{67}/_{56} = 1^{11}/_{56}$

   c) $^{203}/_{120} = 1^{83}/_{120}$

7. a) $\frac{3}{8}$

b) $\frac{1}{12}$

c) $\frac{1}{16}$

8. a) $\frac{37}{32} = 1\frac{5}{32}$

b) $\frac{8}{63}$

c) $\frac{455}{16} = 28\frac{7}{16}$

9. a) $\frac{16}{21}$

b) $\frac{20}{21}$

c) $\frac{40}{21} = 1\frac{19}{21}$

10. a) $\frac{12}{10} = 1\frac{2}{10} = 1\frac{1}{5}$

b) $\frac{14}{24} = \frac{7}{12}$

c) $\frac{35}{24} = 1\frac{11}{24}$

Chapter

2

Decimals

The nurse frequently encounters decimal numbers, because the most commonly used measuring system for medications—the metric system—uses decimal numbers. The nurse also frequently encounters decimal fractions (fractions whose denominators are powers of 10, such as 10, 100, and 1,000). In decimal numbers, the decimal point separates the whole number from the decimal fraction. To the right of the decimal point, each place represents a fraction whose denominator is a power of 10. Each place has a name. From the decimal point to the left, the places include *ones, tens, hundreds, thousands, ten thousands, hundred thousands,* and so on. From the decimal point to the right, the places represent *tenths, hundredths, thousandths, ten thousandths, hundred thousandths,* and so on. (See *Decimal places* for an example.) A nurse rarely encounters decimal fractions beyond the thousandths place.

Decimal places

Based on its relative position to the decimal point, each decimal place represents a power of 10 or a fraction whose denominator is a power of 10, as shown below.

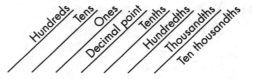

When discussing decimal numbers, use the word *point* in place of the decimal point. For example, you would say the number 3.1 as "three point one." When dealing with money, use the word *and* in place of the decimal point. For example, you would say the price $1.10 as "one dollar and ten cents." When preparing to perform mathematical functions with decimal numbers, eliminate zeros appearing to the right of the decimal point that do not appear between other numbers. However, answers to mathematical calculations and ordered drug dosages always should be written with a zero in front of the decimal point, if no other number appears there, to draw attention to this important symbol and prevent errors.

Once familiar with the basic terms used with decimal fractions, you are ready to review the decimal calculations that a nurse most frequently performs.

Adding decimal fractions

When adding decimal fractions, line up the decimal points vertically. To maintain column alignment, add zeros as placeholders:

Without placeholders	With placeholders
1.34	1.340
.216	0.216
+ 7.1	+ 7.100
8.656	8.656

Without placeholders	With placeholders
9.3	9.300
.604	0.604
+ 2.57	+ 2.570
12.474	12.474

Adding decimal fractions

Add the following decimal fractions. To check your answers, see page 25.

1. 1.31 + 0.4
2. 0.5 + 0.7 + 1.2
3. 5.4 + 2.6 + 0.09
4. 4.1 + 3.03 + 0.4

Subtracting decimal fractions

When subtracting decimal fractions, apply the same rules. Decimal point alignment in a vertical column helps to keep track of the decimal positions. Zeros as placeholders can be helpful:

Without placeholders	With placeholders
5.34	5.340
− .206	− 0.206
5.134	5.134

Without placeholders	With placeholders
12.76	12.760
− .598	− 00.598
12.162	12.162

Subtracting decimal fractions

Subtract the following decimal fractions. To check your answers, see page 25.

1. 4.32 − 3.11
2. 5.75 − 4.03
3. 0.2 − 0.06
4. 1.8 − 0.08

Multiplying decimal fractions

For a multiplication problem with decimal fractions, you do not need to align the decimal points. Just write the problem like any other multiplication problem and leave the decimal points in their original positions. In the final product, the number of decimal places equals the sum of the decimal places in the numbers being multiplied. Count the decimal places starting from the right in the product and place the decimal point, as shown in the examples below:

$$
\begin{array}{r}
6.3 \\
\times \quad 0.65 \\
\hline
4.095
\end{array}
\qquad
\begin{array}{l}
\text{1 decimal place} \\
\text{2 decimal places} \\
\text{3 decimal places in total}
\end{array}
$$

$$
\begin{array}{r}
3.751 \\
\times \quad 8.26 \\
\hline
30.98326
\end{array}
\qquad
\begin{array}{l}
\text{3 decimal places} \\
\text{2 decimal places} \\
\text{5 decimal places in total}
\end{array}
$$

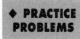
Multiplying decimal fractions

Multiply the following decimal fractions. To check your answers, see page 25.

1. 1.49 × 0.04
2. 0.15 × 3.04
3. 1.31 × 2.07
4. 0.2 × 0.03

Dividing decimal fractions

When dividing decimal fractions, you can place the decimal point if you understand the parts of a division problem. The number to be divided is the *dividend.* The number that divides is the *divisor.* The answer is the *quotient.*

When the divisor is a whole number, place the decimal point in the quotient directly above the dividend's decimal point:

$$
\begin{array}{r}
2.25 \quad \text{quotient} \\
\text{divisor} \quad 3\,\overline{)\,6.75} \quad \text{dividend}
\end{array}
$$

$$
\begin{array}{r}
06.5 \quad \text{quotient} \\
\text{divisor} \quad 15\,\overline{)\,97.5} \quad \text{dividend}
\end{array}
$$

When dividing one decimal fraction by another, move the divisor's decimal point to the right to convert it to a whole number. Then, move the dividend's decimal point the same number of decimal places to the right. After completing the division problem, place the quotient's decimal point directly above the new decimal point in the dividend, as shown in the examples below:

Solve 12.702 ÷ 7.3.

◆ Move the divisor's decimal point one place to the right to make it a whole number.

◆ Move the dividend's decimal point one place to the right.

◆ Place the quotient's decimal point over the new decimal point in the dividend.

$$73. \overline{)127.02}^{\,1.74}$$

Solve 27.234 ÷ 6.56

◆ Move the divisor's decimal point two places to the right to make it a whole number.

◆ Move the dividend's decimal point two places to the right.

◆ Place the quotient's decimal point over the new decimal point in the dividend.

$$656. \overline{)2723.4}^{\,4.15152...\ or\ 4.15}$$

In the second example, the quotient was rounded off because the numbers do not divide evenly. (See "Rounding off decimal fractions" below for a description of this process.)

Dividing decimal fractions

Divide the following fractions, calculating the answers to the nearest thousandth. To check your answers, see page 25.

1. 1.3 ÷ 0.7
2. 1.9 ÷ 3.2
3. 4.1 ÷ 2.05
4. 8.5 ÷ 12

Rounding off decimal fractions

Because most instruments and measuring devices measure accurately only to a tenth or, at most, to a hundredth, the nurse will need to *round off* decimal fractions. Rounding off means converting a long decimal fraction to an appropriate one with fewer decimal places.

To round off a decimal fraction, inspect the number directly to the right of the decimal place to which it will be rounded off. If that number is 5 or greater, then add 1 to the place. For example, to round off 0.746 to the nearest hundredth, check the number directly to the right of the hundredths position: 6. Because 6 is greater than 5, add 1 to the number in the hundredths position (4), which rounds off this decimal fraction to 0.75.

If the number to the right of the selected decimal place is less than 5, then the number stays unchanged. For example, to round off 9.6289 to the nearest tenth, identify the number in the tenths position: 6. Because the number directly to its right (2) is less than 5, the number in the tenths position stays the same and rounding off to the nearest tenth yields 9.6.

◆ **PRACTICE PROBLEMS**

Rounding off decimal fractions

Round off the following decimal fractions to the nearest hundredth. To check your answers, see page 25.

1. 6.4548
2. 2.987
3. 4.123
4. 1.098

Converting common fractions to decimal fractions

Because many measuring devices have metric calibrations, the nurse frequently needs to convert common fractions to decimal fractions. To perform this simple operation, divide the numerator by the denominator and add zeros as place holders, as shown below:

$$\frac{9}{10} = 9 \div 10 = 10\overline{)9.0}^{\;0.9}$$

In another example,

$$\frac{4}{5} = 4 \div 5 = 5\overline{)4.0}^{\;0.8}$$

To convert a mixed number to a decimal fraction, first convert it to an improper fraction, and then divide the numerator by the denominator, as shown below:

$$3\frac{1}{2} = \frac{7}{2} = 7 \div 2 = 3.5$$

Here is another example:

$$7\frac{2}{5} = \frac{37}{5} = 37 \div 5 = 7.4$$

In most cases, you would round off the answer to the nearest hundredth.

◆ **PRACTICE PROBLEMS**

Converting common fractions to decimal fractions

Convert the following common fractions to decimal fractions. To check your answers, see page 25.

1. 3/5
2. 7/10
3. 4¼
4. 6½

Converting decimal fractions to common fractions

At times, you will need to convert a decimal fraction to a common fraction. To do this, you must know the number of decimal places in the decimal fraction, which reflects the number of zeros in the denominator of the common fraction. For example, the decimal fraction 0.65 has two decimal places, so the denominator of its common fraction is 100 (100 has two zeros). To complete the conversion, remove the decimal point from the decimal fraction and use this number as the numerator:

$$0.65 = \frac{65}{100} \text{ (or } \frac{13}{20} \text{ when reduced to the lowest terms)}$$

Mixed decimal numbers can be converted to mixed fractions or improper fractions reduced to the lowest terms, as shown below:

$$3.25 = 3^{25}/_{100} = 3^{1}/_{4} = {}^{13}/_{4}$$

◆ PRACTICE PROBLEMS	**Converting decimal fractions to common fractions**

Convert the following decimal fractions to common fractions. To check your answers, see page 26.

1. 0.80
2. 0.45
3. 3.15
4. 6.50

Review problems

Calculate the solutions to the following questions about decimals. To check your answers, see page 26.

1. In the following decimal fractions, what number is in the tenths place?

   a) 4.035

   b) 1.2058

   c) 9.677

2. Round off the following decimal fractions to the nearest hundredth.

   a) 7.245

   b) 10.2467

   c) 0.952

3. Add the following decimal fractions.

   a) 0.345 + 9.9

   b) 6.2 + 6.798 + 4.06

   c) 0.455 + 0.04 + 8.97

4. Subtract the following decimal fractions.

   a) 9.005 − 0.04

   b) 3.75 − 0.024

   c) 2.5 − 0.003

5. Multiply the following decimal fractions.

   a) 5.4 × 0.034

   b) 4.9 × 10.203

   c) 7.1 × 0.6

6. Convert the following common fractions to decimals.

   a) ³/₁₀

   b) 4½

7. Convert the following decimal fractions to common fractions.
- a) 0.75
- b) 0.666
- c) 2.83

Answers to practice problems

◆ Adding decimal fractions
1. 1.71
2. 2.4
3. 8.09
4. 7.53

◆ Subtracting decimal fractions
1. 1.21
2. 1.72
3. 0.14
4. 1.72

◆ Multiplying decimal fractions
1. 0.0596
2. 0.456
3. 2.7117
4. 0.006

◆ Dividing decimal fractions
1. 1.857
2. 0.594
3. 2
4. 0.708

◆ Rounding off decimal fractions
1. 6.45
2. 2.99
3. 4.12
4. 1.10

◆ Converting common fractions to decimal fractions
1. 0.60
2. 0.70
3. 4.25
4. 6.50

◆ *Converting decimal fractions to common fractions*

1. $^{80}/_{100} = ^4/_5$

2. $^{45}/_{100} = ^9/_{20}$

3. $^{315}/_{100} = 3\ ^{15}/_{100} = 3\ ^3/_{20}$

4. $^{650}/_{100} = 6\ ^{50}/_{100} = 6\ ^1/_2$

Answers to review problems

1. a) 0
   b) 2
   c) 6

2. a) 7.25
   b) 10.25
   c) 0.95

3. a) 10.245
   b) 17.058
   c) 9.465

4. a) 8.965
   b) 3.726
   c) 2.497

5. a) 0.1836
   b) 49.9947
   c) 4.26

6. a) $^3/_{10} = 3 \div 10 = 0.3$
   b) $4^1/_2 = ^9/_2 = 9 \div 2 = 4.5$

7. a) $^3/_4$
   b) $^2/_3$
   c) $2\ ^{83}/_{100}$

Chapter

3

◆

Percentages

Percentages represent an alternative way to express fractions and numerical relationships. A common term, *percentage* means any quantity stated as the proportion per hundred and is expressed by a percent sign (%), which means "for every hundred." This symbol may be used with a whole number (10%), a mixed number (12½%), a decimal number (0.9%), or a fraction number (¼%). In nursing, you need to be able to convert freely from percentages to decimal and common fractions, and from these fractions to percentages.

Converting percentages to decimal fractions

To change a percentage to a decimal fraction, multiply the number in the percentage by ¹⁄₁₀₀, or 0.01. For example, you would convert 72% to a decimal fraction like this: $72 \times 0.01 = 0.72$. A simpler conversion technique is to remove the percent sign and move the decimal point two places to the left:

Convert 15% to a decimal fraction.
♦ Remove the percent sign.

$$15$$

♦ Move the decimal point two places to the left to obtain the decimal fraction.

$$0.15$$

Convert 6.25% to a decimal fraction.
♦ Remove the percent sign.

$$6.25$$

♦ Move the decimal point two places to the left to obtain the decimal fraction.

$$0.0625$$

◆ **PRACTICE PROBLEMS**

Converting percentages to decimal fractions

Convert the following percentages to decimal fractions. To check your answers, see page 34.

1. 34%
2. 21%
3. 1.3%

    4. 76%

    5. 0.97%

Converting percentages to common fractions

To convert a percentage to a common fraction, follow these three steps. First, change the percentage to a decimal fraction by removing the percent sign and moving the decimal point two places to the left. Second, convert the decimal fraction to a common fraction with the appropriate denominator. (This will be a factor of 10.) Third, reduce the fraction to its lowest terms. The following examples demonstrate this three-step process:

Convert 25% to a common fraction.

◆ Convert by removing the percent sign and moving the decimal point two places to the left.

$$0.25$$

◆ Convert the decimal fraction to a common fraction, using 100 as the denominator because 0.25 has two decimal places.

$$\frac{25}{100}$$

◆ Reduce the common fraction to the lowest terms.

$$\frac{1}{4}$$

Convert 37.5% to a common fraction.

◆ Convert by removing the percent sign and moving the decimal point two places to the left.

$$0.375$$

◆ Convert the decimal fraction to a common fraction, using 1,000 as the denominator because 0.375 has three decimal places.

$$\frac{375}{1,000}$$

◆ Reduce the common fraction to the lowest terms.

$$\frac{3}{8}$$

◆ **PRACTICE PROBLEMS**

Converting percentages to common fractions

Convert the following percentages to common fractions. To check your answers, see page 34.

    1. 36%

    2. 2.45%

    3. 76%

    4. 1.1%

    5. 9.85%

Converting decimal fractions to percentages

To change a decimal fraction to a percentage, reverse the process you used to convert a percentage to a decimal fraction. Move the decimal point two places to the right and add a percent sign:

Convert 0.33 to a percentage.

◆ Move the decimal point two places to the right.

33

◆ Add a percent sign to obtain the percentage.

33%

Convert 0.125 to a percentage.

◆ Move the decimal point two places to the right.

12.5

◆ Add a percent sign to obtain the percentage.

12.5%

◆ **PRACTICE PROBLEMS**

Converting decimal fractions to percentages

Convert the following decimal fractions to percentages. To check your answers, see page 34.

1. 0.11
2. 0.37
3. 2.5
4. 0.019
5. 0.789

Converting common fractions to percentages

Converting any common fraction to a percentage involves two simple steps. First, convert the fraction to a decimal by treating it as a division problem and dividing the numerator by the denominator. (A handheld calculator makes this part of the conversion particularly easy. See *Conversions by calculator*).

Convert ⅜ to a percentage.

◆ Convert ⅜ to a decimal fraction by dividing 8 into 3.

0.375

◆ Convert the decimal fraction to a percentage by moving the decimal point two places to the right and adding the percent sign.

37.5%

Convert ⅔ to a percentage.

◆ Convert ⅔ to a decimal fraction by dividing 3 into 2. (Round off to two decimal places.)

0.666 = 0.67

◆ Convert the decimal fraction to a percentage by moving the decimal point two places to the right and adding the percent sign.

67%

Conversions by calculator

A handheld calculator can simplify converting a common fraction to a decimal fraction. For example, to convert a mixed number, such as 5⅝, to a decimal fraction, convert it to an improper fraction (⁴⁵⁄₈) and follow these steps.

1. Enter the numerator (45).

2. Press ÷.

3. Enter the denominator (8).

4. Press = to obtain the converted number (5.625).

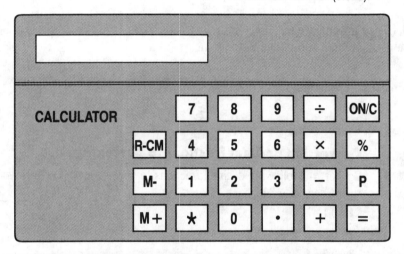

◆ **PRACTICE PROBLEMS**

Converting common fractions to percentages

Convert the following common fractions to percentages. To check your answers, see page 34.

1. ⁵⁄₁₆

2. ⅛

3. ⅞

4. ³⁄₇

5. ⅓

Solving percentage problems

To solve percentage problems, the nurse must first understand the three different types of calculations.

1. Find which number is a certain percent of another number.

2. Find what percent one number is of another.

3. Find which number is a specified percentage of another number.

Solving each type can be made easier by following a few simple rules. The question "What is 15% of 300?" is an example of the first type. To solve it, change the word *of* to a multiplication sign.

Then convert 15% to a decimal fraction by removing the percent sign and moving the decimal point two places to the left. Then multiply as shown below:

What is 15% of 300?
♦ In this case, *of* means multiply. Restate the question as a multiplication problem.

$$15\% \times 300 = \underline{\hspace{2cm}}$$

♦ Convert 15% to a decimal fraction by removing the percent sign and moving the decimal point two places to the left.

$$0.15$$

♦ Multiply to solve for the percent.

$$\begin{array}{r} 0.15 \\ \times\ \ 300 \\ \hline 45 \end{array}$$

What is 8% of 175?
♦ Restate the question as a multiplication problem.

$$8\% \times 175 = \underline{\hspace{2cm}}$$

♦ Convert 8% to a decimal fraction removing the percent sign and moving the decimal point two places to the left.

$$0.08$$

♦ Multiply to solve for percent.

$$\begin{array}{r} 175 \\ \times\ \ 0.08 \\ \hline 14 \end{array}$$

To find what percent one number is of another, change the word *of* to a division sign, and divide. The first number becomes the dividend; the second becomes the divisor. Then move the decimal point in the quotient two places to the right.

25 is what percent of 200?
♦ In this case, *of* means divide. Restate the question as a division problem.

$$200 \overline{\smash)25.00} \quad \overset{0.125}{}$$

♦ Move the decimal point in the quotient two places to the right.

$$0.125 = 12.5$$

♦ Add a percent sign.

$$12.5\%$$

36 is what percent of 144?
♦ Restate the question as a division problem.

$$144 \overline{\smash)36.00} \quad \overset{0.25}{}$$

♦ Move the decimal point in the quotient two places to the right.

$$0.25 = 25$$

♦ Add a percent sign.

$$25\%$$

This type of problem also can be expressed in this way:

What percent of 16 is 8?
◆ Restate the question as a division problem.

$$16\overline{)8.00}^{\,0.50}$$

◆ Move the decimal point two places to the right.

$$0.50 = 50$$

◆ Add a percent sign.

$$50\%$$

What percent of 250 is 8?
◆ Restate the question as a division problem.

$$250\overline{)8.000}^{\,0.032}$$

◆ Move the decimal point two places to the right.

$$0.032 = 3.2$$

◆ Add a percent sign.

$$3.2\%$$

When the divisor does not divide exactly into the dividend, state the answer as a mixed number. Do this by leaving the remainder after two decimal places as a common fraction, as shown below:

2 is what percent of 9?
◆ Restate the question as a division problem, leaving the remainder after two places as a common fraction.

$$9\overline{)2.00}^{\,0.22\frac{2}{9}}$$

◆ Move the decimal point in the quotient two places to the right.

$$0.22\tfrac{2}{9} = 22\tfrac{2}{9}$$

◆ Add a percent sign.

$$22\tfrac{2}{9}\%$$

11 is what percent of 15?
◆ Restate the question as a division problem, leaving the remainder after two places as a common fraction.

$$15\overline{)11.00}^{\,0.73\frac{5}{15}\text{ or }.73\frac{1}{3}}$$

◆ Move the decimal point in the quotient two places to the right.

$$0.73\tfrac{1}{3} = 73\tfrac{1}{3}$$

◆ Add a percent sign.

$$73\tfrac{1}{3}\%$$

The third type of problem, finding which number another is a specified percentage of, also is a division problem. The number expressed as a percentage must be converted to a decimal fraction by moving the decimal point two places to the left. That decimal fraction then becomes the divisor.

70% of what number is 42?

* Convert the percentage to a decimal fraction by removing the percent sign and moving the decimal point two places to the left.

$$70\% = 0.70$$

* Divide the decimal fraction into the number. (In other words, divide the number by the decimal fraction.)

$$070. \overline{)4200.} \quad \overset{60.}{}$$

60% of what number is 210?

* Convert the percentage to a decimal fraction by removing the percent sign and moving the decimal point two places to the left.

$$60\% = 0.60$$

* Divide the decimal fraction into the number.

$$.60 \overline{)210} = 60 \overline{)21000} \quad \overset{350}{}$$

◆ **PRACTICE PROBLEMS**

Solving percentage problems

Solve the following problems to determine percentages. To check your answers, see pages 34 and 35.

1. What is 16% of the following numbers?
   a) 242
   b) 108
   c) 79
   d) 10

2. 25 is what percent of the following numbers?
   a) 25
   b) 300

3. 70% of what number is 28?

4. 70% of what number is 7?

5. 30% of what number is 90?

Review problems

Solve the following percentage problems. To check your answers, see page 35.

1. What is 25% of 200?

2. 0.125 is what percent of 0.25?

3. What is 11.3% of 25?

4. ¼ is what percent of ½?

5. What is 5% of 1,000?

6. 250 is what percent of 1,000?

7. What is 0.9% of 1,000?

8. 30 is what percent of 50?

9. What is 0.45% of 500?

10. 1⅓ is what percent of 2?

11. Convert the following common fractions to percentages.

   a) ⅝

   b) ⅓

   c) ⁷⁄₁₀

Answers to practice problems

◆ **Converting percentages to decimal fractions**

1. 0.34

2. 0.21

3. 0.013

4. 0.76

5. 0.0097

◆ **Converting percentages to common fractions**

1. ³⁶⁄₁₀₀ = ⁹⁄₂₅

2. ²⁴⁵⁄₁₀,₀₀₀ = ⁴⁹⁄₂,₀₀₀

3. ⁷⁶⁄₁₀₀ = ³⁸⁄₅₀ = ¹⁹⁄₂₅

4. ¹¹⁄₁,₀₀₀

5. ⁹⁸⁵⁄₁₀,₀₀₀ = ¹⁹⁷⁄₂,₀₀₀

◆ **Converting decimal fractions to percentages**

1. 11%

2. 37%

3. 250%

4. 1.9%

5. 78.9%

◆ **Converting common fractions to percentages**

1. 31.25%

2. 12.5%

3. 116.67%

4. 42.86%

5. 33.33%

◆ **Solving percentage problems**

1. a) 38.72

   b) 17.28

   c) 12.64

   d) 1.6

2. a) 100%

   b) 8.3%

3. 40

4. 10

5. 300

Answers to review problems

1. 50

2. 50%

3. 2.825 = 2.8

4. 50%

5. 50

6. 25%

7. 9

8. 60%

9. 2.25

10. 66.66 = 66.7%

11. a) 62.5%

   b) 33⅓%

   c) 70%

Chapter

4

Ratios, Fractions, and Proportions

Ratios and fractions are mathematical expressions that describe the relationship between numbers. They both state how numbers relate to each other. However, ratios use a colon between the numbers in the relationship, such as 2 : 5, whereas fractions use a slash, such as ⅖. Proportions are statements of equality between two ratios, such as 2 : 5 :: 4 : 10, or between two fractions, such as ⅖ = ⁴⁄₁₀.

When calculating dosages, you'll use ratios, fractions, and proportions frequently. You'll also find them useful for solving many other related problems, such as calculating I.V. infusion rates, converting weights between systems of measurement, and (in specialty settings) performing oxygenation and hemodynamic calculations. But before you can put ratios, fractions, and proportions into use, you need to know how to develop and express them appropriately.

Expressing numerical relationships as ratios and fractions

A *ratio* and a *fraction* are numerical ways to compare items. If a hospital hires three ancillary workers for every professional hired, then the number of ancillary workers to professionals is 3 to 1. This can be written as the ratio 3 : 1 or as the fraction ¾. In a ratio or fraction, pay attention to which item is mentioned first. For example, the number of ancillary workers to professionals is 3 to 1, but the number of professionals to ancillary workers is 1 to 3, which can be written as 1 : 3 or ⅓. Here are a few more examples.

If a hospital's critical care area requires one registered nurse for every two patients, then the relationship of registered nurses to patients is 1 to 2. You can express this relationship with the ratio 1 : 2 or with the fraction ½.

In medication administration, you frequently need to use ratios and fractions to express the dosage of medication per capsule, tablet, or volume of solution. For example, one tablet contains 325 mg of acetaminophen. By using a ratio, you can express this as 1 tablet : 325 mg. By using a fraction, you can describe it as 1 tablet/325 mg.

Expressing numerical relationships as ratios and fractions

Express each of the following statements as a ratio and as a fraction. To check your answers, see page 39.

1. In our department, 35 staff members are supervised by one nurse manager.
2. One tablet of digoxin contains 0.125 mg.
3. Twelve bags of I.V. fluid come in one case.
4. On the medical-surgical floor, two teams of nurses care for 35 patients.

Expressing proportions with ratios

Simply speaking, a *proportion* is a set of two equal ratios or fractions. When using ratios to express a proportion, you separate the ratios with double colons. For example, if the ratio of ancillary workers to professionals is 3 : 1, then this would mean six ancillary workers are available for every two professionals. This proportion could be written as:

3 workers : 1 professional :: 6 workers : 2 professionals

or

3 : 1 :: 6 : 2

Here's another example. If the department has one registered nurse for every two patients, you could express this as the ratio 1 : 2. You could also say that this equals a ratio of three registered nurses for every six patients. In a proportion, you can express this relationship with ratios as follows:

1 RN : 2 patients :: 3 RNs : 6 patients

or

1 : 2 :: 3 : 6

Now suppose you have one tablet that contains 325 mg of acetaminophen. You could state this as the ratio 1 tablet : 325 mg, which equals the ratio 2 tablets : 650 mg. This proportion can be expressed with ratios as follows:

1 tablet : 325 mg :: 2 tablets : 650 mg

or

1 : 325 :: 2 : 650

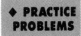

Expressing proportions with ratios

Express the following proportions using ratios. To check your answers, see page 39.

1. The school of nursing has one clinical instructor for every five students. Therefore, a staff of five clinical instructors should teach 25 nursing students.
2. A container holds 8 mg of a drug in 1 ml. So there must be 4 mg of the drug in 0.5 ml.
3. A nurse works 10 days in one pay period, which means that the nurse works 20 days in two pay periods.

Expressing proportions with fractions

Any proportion that can be expressed with ratios can also be expressed with fractions. Using the examples above, let's see the same data expressed with fractions. If a department has three ancillary workers for every one professional, that means it has six ancillary workers for every two professionals. Using fractions, you could write this proportion as:

3 workers/1 professional = 6 workers/2 professionals

or

$\frac{3}{1} = \frac{6}{2}$

In the department with one registered nurse for every two patients (which equals a ratio of three registered nurses for every six patients), you could express this relationship in a proportion with fractions as:

1 RN/2 patients = 3 RNs/6 patients

or

$\frac{1}{2} = \frac{3}{6}$

When one tablet contains 325 mg of acetaminophen and two tablets contain 650 mg, the proportion can be expressed with fractions as:

325 mg/1 tablet = 650 mg/2 tablets

or

$\frac{325}{1} = \frac{650}{2}$

◆ **PRACTICE PROBLEMS**

Expressing proportions with fractions

Express the following proportions using fractions. To check your answers, see page 39.

1. One tablet contains 30 mg of a drug. Therefore, four tablets contain 120 mg of the drug.

2. A vial holds 125 mg of a drug in 10 ml. So two vials hold 250 mg of the drug in 20 ml.

3. A bottle label states that it contains 10 mg of a drug in 5 ml, which equals 5 mg of the drug in 2.5 ml.

Review problems

Solve the following problems involving ratios, fractions, and proportions. To check your answers, see page 39.

1. Rewrite the ratio 3 : 8 as a fraction.

2. Use fractions to express the following proportion: The department has five patients to one LPN, or ten patients to two LPNs.

3. Use ratios to express the following proportion: $\frac{3}{36} = \frac{1}{12}$.

4. Is the following statement a true proportion? 4 : 5 :: 8 : 12

5. Write this numerical relationship as a fraction: 5 mg in 10 ml.

6. Write this numerical relationship as a ratio: 100 mg in 20 ml.

7. Express the following proportion using ratios: 100 mg in 20 ml = 200 mg in 40 ml.

8. Express the following proportion using fractions: 1 : 5 :: 2 : 10.

Answers to practice problems

◆ Expressing numerical relationships as ratios and fractions

1. $35:1$ or $^{35}/_1$
2. $1:0.125$ or $^{1}/_{0.125}$
3. $12:1$ or $^{12}/_1$
4. $2:35$ or $^{2}/_{35}$

◆ Expressing proportions with ratios

1. 1 instructor : 5 students :: 5 instructors : 25 students or $1:5::5:25$
2. 8 mg : 1 ml :: 4 mg : 0.5 ml or $8:1::4:0.5$
3. 10 days : 1 pay period :: 20 days : 2 pay periods or $10:1::20:2$

◆ Expressing proportions with fractions

1. 1 tablet/30 mg = 4 tablets/120 mg or $^{1}/_{30} = {^{4}/_{120}}$
2. 125 mg/10 ml = 250 mg/20 ml or $^{125}/_{10} = {^{250}/_{20}}$
3. 10 mg/5 ml = 5 mg/2.5 ml or $^{10}/_5 = {^{5}/_{2.5}}$

Answers to review problems

1. $^{3}/_8$
2. 5 patients/1 LPN = 10 patients/2 LPNs or $^{5}/_1 = {^{10}/_2}$
3. $3:36::1:12$
4. No, because the ratios are not equal.
5. 5 mg/10 ml or $^{5}/_{10}$
6. 100 mg : 20 ml or $100:20$
7. 100 mg : 20 ml :: 200 mg : 40 ml
8. $^{1}/_5 = {^{2}/_{10}}$

Chapter

Equations to Find the Value of X

As you saw in Chapter 4, a proportion is a set of two equal ratios or fractions. In a proportion, if one ratio or fraction is complete and the other is incomplete, you can solve for X to determine the value of the unknown quantity.

The ability to find the value of X is vital in nursing—especially in dosage calculations. For example, suppose a physician orders a drug for a patient, but the drug isn't available in the dosage strength ordered. In this case, you must find the value of X, which is the amount of the drug to administer.

Before using proportions to determine the value of X, let's review how to find X by solving equations with whole numbers and fractions.

Solving equations with common fractions

The steps in solving common-fraction equations form the basis for solving other types of simple equations to find the value of X. Just follow the steps below.

Solve for X in the following common-fraction equation.
$$X = \frac{3}{50} \times \frac{1}{3}$$

◆ First, multiply the numerators.
$$3 \times 1 = 3$$

◆ Next, multiply the denominators.
$$50 \times 3 = 150$$

◆ Restate the equation with this new information.
$$X = \frac{3 \times 1}{50 \times 3} = \frac{3}{150}$$

◆ Reduce the fraction by dividing the numerator and denominator by the highest common denominator (3).
$$X = \frac{1}{50}$$

◆ Because most dosage calculations require your answer to be in decimal form, convert your answer to a decimal fraction. (As needed, round your answer to the nearest tenth or hundredth.)
$$X = 0.02$$

◆ PRACTICE PROBLEMS

Solving equations with common fractions

Solve for X in the following equations with common fractions. Express your answers both as common fractions and as decimal fractions. To check your answers, see page 47.

1. $X = \frac{2}{3} \times \frac{5}{8}$
2. $X = \frac{1}{5} \times \frac{3}{9}$
3. $X = \frac{23}{29} \times \frac{11}{17}$
4. $X = \frac{1}{2} \times \frac{3}{1,000}$
5. $X = \frac{28}{29} \times \frac{4}{27}$

Solving equations with whole numbers

To solve whole-number equations to find the value of X, use the following steps.

Solve for X in the following whole-number equation.

$$X = \frac{30}{20} \times 2$$

◆ First, convert the whole number 2 into the fraction $\frac{2}{1}$. (Remember that you can express any whole number as the numerator of a fraction whose denominator is 1.)

$$X = \frac{30}{20} \times \frac{2}{1}$$

◆ To simplify the rest of the math, reduce the fraction $\frac{30}{20}$ by its highest common denominator, which is 10.

$$X = \frac{3}{2} \times \frac{2}{1}$$

◆ Multiply the numbers as you would in any common fraction. Simply multiply the numerators (3 × 2) and the denominators (2 × 1).

$$X = \frac{3 \times 2}{1 \times 2} = \frac{6}{2}$$

◆ Reduce the answer. Because the answer is an improper fraction in this example, divide the numerator 6 by the denominator 2.

$$X = 3$$

Here is another example, using a whole number in an equation.

$$X = \frac{25,000}{400,000} \times 4$$

◆ Convert the whole number 4 to a fraction.

$$X = \frac{25,000}{400,000} \times \frac{4}{1}$$

◆ Reduce the fraction $\frac{25,000}{400,000}$ by its highest common denominator, 25,000.

$$X = \frac{1}{16} \times \frac{4}{1}$$

◆ Multiply the numerators (1 × 4) and the denominators (16 × 1).

$$X = \frac{1 \times 4}{16 \times 1} = \frac{4}{16}$$

◆ Reduce the answer.

$$X = \frac{1}{4}$$

◆ Convert your answer to a decimal fraction.

$$X = 0.25$$

<table>
<tr><td>

◆ PRACTICE PROBLEMS

</td><td>

Solving equations with whole numbers

Solve for X in the following equations with whole numbers. To check your answers, see page 47.

</td></tr>
</table>

1. $X = {}^{125}\!/_{500} \times 3$
2. $X = {}^{75}\!/_{25} \times 2$
3. $X = {}^{5,000}\!/_{100,000} \times 4$
4. $X = 6 \times {}^{15}\!/_{18}$
5. $X = {}^{12}\!/_{8} \times 15$

Solving equations with decimal fractions

To solve for X in equations with decimal fractions, follow similar steps to the ones you used above.

Solve for X in the following decimal fraction equation.

$$X = {}^{0.03}\!/_{0.05} \times 2$$

◆ First, remove the decimal points from the fraction. To do this, move them both two spaces to the right.

$$X = {}^{3}\!/_{5} \times 2$$

◆ Next, convert the whole number 2 into a fraction whose denominator is 1.

$$X = {}^{3}\!/_{5} \times {}^{2}\!/_{1}$$

◆ Then, multiply the numerators (3 × 2) and the denominators (5 × 1) and restate the equation.

$$X = \frac{3 \times 2}{5 \times 1} = \frac{6}{5}$$

◆ Finally, reduce the answer and convert it to decimal form.

$$X = 1.2$$

Here's another example that uses decimal fractions to solve for X.

$$X = {}^{0.125}\!/_{0.25} \times 0.5$$

◆ First, remove the decimal points. To do this with the fraction on the left, move the decimal points three spaces to the right.

$$X = {}^{125}\!/_{250} \times 0.5$$

◆ Next, convert the number 0.5 into a fraction whose denominator is 1.

$$X = {}^{125}\!/_{250} \times {}^{0.5}\!/_{1}$$

◆ Then, multiply the numerators (125 × 0.5) and the denominators (250 × 1) and restate the equation.

$$X = \frac{125 \times 0.5}{250 \times 1} = \frac{6.25}{250}$$

◆ Finally, reduce the answer and convert it to decimal form.

$$X = 0.25$$

◆ PRACTICE PROBLEMS	**Solving equations with decimal fractions**

Solve for X in the following equations with decimal fractions. To check your answers, see pages 47 and 48.

1. $X = {}^{0.05}\!/_{0.02} \times 3$
2. $X = {}^{0.75}\!/_{0.25} \times 5$
3. $X = {}^{0.125}\!/_{0.625} \times .5$
4. $X = {}^{0.33}\!/_{0.11} \times 6$
5. $X = {}^{0.04}\!/_{0.05} \times 4$

Solving proportion problems with ratios

When a proportion is written with ratios, as in $3:1::6:2$, the proportion's outer (or end) numbers (3 and 2) are the *extremes;* its inner (or middle) numbers (1 and 6) are the *means.* In such a proportion, the product of the means equals the product of the extremes. In this case, $1 \times 6 = 3 \times 2$. This principle lets you solve for any one of four unknown parts in a proportion, as shown below:

Solve for X in this proportion.

$$6:X = 3:8$$

◆ Rewrite the problem to multiply the means and the extremes.

$$3 \times X = 8 \times 6$$

◆ Obtain the products of the means and extremes in an equation.

$$3X = 48$$

◆ Solve for X by dividing both sides by 3.

$$\frac{3X}{3} = \frac{48}{3}$$

◆ Find X.

$$X = 16$$

◆ Restate the proportion in ratios.

$$3:8::6:16$$

Solve for X in this proportion.

$$25:40::5:X$$

◆ Rewrite the problem to multiply the means and the extremes.

$$25 \times X = 40 \times 5$$

◆ Obtain the products of the means and extremes in an equation.

$$25X = 200$$

◆ Solve for X by dividing both sides by 25.

$$\frac{25X}{25} = \frac{200}{25}$$

◆ Find X.

$$X = 8$$

◆ Restate the proportion in ratios.

$$25:40::5:8$$

Golden Rules

In a proportion with ratios, the product of the **m**eans (numbers in the **m**iddle) equals the product of the **e**xtremes (numbers on the **e**nds).

◆ **PRACTICE PROBLEMS**

Solving proportion problems with ratios

Solve for X in the following proportions with ratios. To check your answers, see page 48.

1. $4:8::8:X$
2. $3:6::6:X$
3. $X:12::6:24$
4. $10:20::X:40$
5. $5:25::15:X$

Solving proportion problems with fractions

In a proportion expressed as a fraction, *cross products* are equal. In other words, the numerator on the equation's left side multiplied by the denominator on the equation's right side equals the denominator on the equation's left side multiplied by the numerator on the equation's right side. Using the cross products of a proportion, the nurse can solve for any one of four unknown parts.

Solve for X in this proportion.

$$\frac{5}{2} = \frac{X}{4}$$

◆ Rewrite the problem to multiply the cross products.

$$2 \times X = 5 \times 4$$

◆ Obtain the cross products.

$$2X = 20$$

◆ Solve for X by dividing both sides by 2.

$$\frac{2X}{2} = \frac{20}{2}$$

◆ Find X.

$$X = 10$$

◆ Restate the proportion in fractions.

$$\frac{5}{2} = \frac{10}{4}$$

Solve for X in the following proportion.

$$\frac{X}{3} = \frac{15}{9}$$

◆ Rewrite the problem to multiply the cross products.

$$3 \times 15 = X \times 9$$

◆ Obtain the cross products.

$$45 = 9X$$

◆ Solve for X by dividing both sides by 9.

$$\frac{45}{9} = \frac{9X}{9}$$

◆ Find X.

$$5 = X$$

◆ Restate the proportion in fractions.

$$\frac{5}{3} = \frac{15}{9}$$

◆ PRACTICE PROBLEMS

Solving proportion problems with fractions

Solve for X in the following proportions with fractions. To check your answers, see page 48.

1. $\dfrac{4}{3} = \dfrac{X}{6}$

2. $\dfrac{12}{25} = \dfrac{X}{50}$

3. $\dfrac{15}{X} = \dfrac{30}{120}$

4. $\dfrac{X}{7} = \dfrac{3}{21}$

5. $\dfrac{3}{4} = \dfrac{9}{X}$

Setting up proportions

When setting up a proportion, place the known ratio on one side of the double colon and unknown ratio on the other side, making certain that the similar parts of each ratio are in the same position relative to the colon.

How much salt should be added to one quart to make a solution that contains ½ teaspoon salt for every 8 ounces of water?

◆ Set up the proportion so that similar parts of each ratio are in the same position.

½ tsp salt : 8 oz water :: X tsp salt : 32 oz (1 qt) water

◆ Solve for X.

$$8X = \text{½} \times 32$$
$$8X = 16$$
$$\frac{8X}{8} = \frac{16}{8}$$
$$X = 2 \text{ tsp salt}$$

◆ If you set up the proportion with fractions, follow the same rule: Place similar parts of each fraction in the same position in the fractions.

$$\frac{\frac{1}{2} \text{ tsp salt}}{8 \text{ oz water}} = \frac{X \text{ tsp salt}}{32 \text{ oz water}}$$

◆ Solve for X.

$$8X = \frac{1}{2} \times 32$$
$$8X = 16$$
$$X = 2 \text{ tsp salt}$$

◆ **PRACTICE PROBLEMS**

Setting up proportions

Set up the following proportions and solve for X. To check your answers, see page 48.

1. If one ancillary worker is required for every six patients, how many workers are needed for 30 patients?

2. How much hydrogen peroxide should you add to 1,000 ml of water to make a solution that contains 50 ml of hydrogen peroxide for every 100 ml of water?

3. If the school of nursing requires one nursing instructor for every eight students, how many instructors are needed for 48 students?

4. One case of I.V. fluid holds 20 bags. If the medical-surgical floor receives six cases, how many bags of I.V. fluid does it have?

Review problems

Solve for X in the following problems. To check your answers, see pages 48 and 49.

1. $X = \frac{2}{7} \times \frac{3}{5}$

2. $X = \frac{3}{50} \times 6$

3. $X = \frac{0.125}{0.25} \times 2$

4. $X = \frac{0.4}{0.02} \times 0.8$

5. $X : 4 :: 3 : 5$

6. $X : 100 :: 100 : 1,000$

7. $\frac{1}{4} : 1 :: \frac{1}{2} : X$

8. $X : 0.25 :: 0.5 : 1$

9. $3 : 10 :: 12 : X$

10. $5 : 6 :: 7 : X$

11. $3 : X :: 12 : 36$

12. $7 : 1 :: 49 : X$

13. $2.2 : 3.5 :: 1 : X$

14. $\dfrac{X}{55} = \dfrac{1}{2.2}$

15. $\dfrac{X}{75} = \dfrac{0.5}{50}$

16. $\dfrac{X}{100} = \dfrac{5}{125}$

17. $\dfrac{\frac{1}{2}}{0.5} = \dfrac{\frac{1}{4}}{X}$

18. $\dfrac{80}{10} = \dfrac{60}{X}$

19. $\dfrac{6}{7} = \dfrac{24}{X}$

20. $\dfrac{X}{7} = \dfrac{5}{35}$

21. How much salt should you add to 16 ounces of water to make a solution that contains 1 teaspoon of salt for every 8 ounces of water?

22. If a vial has 50 mg of a drug in 5 ml, how many milligrams of the drug exist in 15 ml?

23. A 36-bed unit requires six staff members for each shift. If an 18-bed unit has the same staffing ratio, how many staff members does it need for each shift?

Answers to practice problems

◆ Solving equations with common fractions

1. $X = {}^{10}\!/_{24} = {}^{5}\!/_{12}$ or $X = 0.42$

2. $X = {}^{3}\!/_{45} = {}^{1}\!/_{15}$ or $X = 0.066$, rounded to 0.067

3. $X = {}^{253}\!/_{493}$ or $X = 0.51$

4. $X = {}^{3}\!/_{2,000}$ or $X = 0.002$

5. $X = {}^{112}\!/_{783}$ or $X = 0.14$

◆ Solving equations with whole numbers

1. 0.75

2. 6

3. 0.2

4. 5

5. 22.5

◆ Solving equations with decimal fractions

1. 7.5

2. 15

3. 0.1

4. 18

5. 3.2

♦ *Solving proportion problems with ratios*

1. 16

2. 12

3. 3

4. 20

5. 75

♦ *Solving proportion problems with fractions*

1. 8

2. 24

3. 60

4. 1

5. 12

♦ *Setting up proportions*

1. $1 : 6 :: X : 30$, in which $X = 5$ workers

2. $X : 1,000 :: 50 : 100$, in which $X = 500$ ml hydrogen peroxide

3. $1 : 8 :: X : 48$, in which $X = 6$ instructors

4. $1 : 20 :: 6 : X$, in which $X = 120$ bags

Answers to review problems

1. $X = \frac{6}{35}$ or 0.17

2. $X = \frac{18}{50}$ or 0.36

3. $X = \frac{0.25}{0.25}$ or 1

4. $X = \frac{0.32}{0.02}$ or 16

5. $2\frac{2}{5} = 2.4$

6. 10

7. 2

8. 0.125

9. 40

10. $8\frac{2}{5} = 8.4$

11. 9

12. 7

13. $1.59 = 1.6$

14. 25

15. 0.75
16. 4
17. 0.25
18. 7.5
19. 28
20. 1
21. X : 16 :: 1 : 8, in which X = 2 tsp
22. 50 : 5 :: X : 15, in which X = 150 mg
23. 36 : 6 :: 18 : X, in which X = 3 staff members

UNIT 2

◆

Systems of Drug Measurement

The major systems used for drug weights and measures are the metric, apothecaries', household, avoirdupois, unit, and milliequivalent (mEq) systems. This unit describes each of these systems, their basic units of measurement, and how to make conversions within each system and among different systems. It also provides patient situations, practice problems, and review problems.

Although the metric system is the most widely used system of drug weights and measures, you'll need to be familiar with all of the systems. In clinical practice, you'll usually administer drugs that are measured in units and mEqs.

Rarely, you may see orders for drugs measured in the apothecaries' system. Such orders typically are for older drugs and are written by physicians who were trained to use this system. Until the metric system totally replaces the apothecaries' system (as recommended by the United States Pharmacopeial Convention), you'll need to check the pharmacist's conversion to the measurement system in which the drug is supplied.

When caring for pediatric or home care patients, you'll need to handle conversions to the household and sometimes avoirdupois systems. These systems are familiar to most patients and are the ones they're most likely to use at home.

Chapter

6

Metric System

In school and college science courses, students usually learn the metric system, the measurement system used by most nations. Because the metric system is based on powers of 10, it offers several advantages over other measurement systems: it eliminates common fractions, simplifies the calculation of larger or smaller units, and simplifies the calculation of drug dosages.

Units of measurement

The first step to understanding the metric system is to become familiar with its three basic units of measurement: the meter, liter, and gram.

The *meter* (m) is the basic unit of length. The *liter* (L) is the basic unit of volume, representing ¹/₁₀ of a cubic meter. The *gram* (g) is the basic unit of weight, representing the weight of one cubic centimeter of water at 4° C.

All other units of measure are based on the meter, liter, and gram. In fact, the names of these basic units are incorporated in the names of related units, which makes it easy to determine what type of unit you're measuring. For example, a kilo*gram* and a milli*gram* are both units of weight.

To make measurements in the metric system, you must use the device that is appropriate to the unit of measurement. (See *Metric measurement devices,* page 52, for illustrations.)

 PRACTICE PROBLEMS

Units of measurement

For the following metric units, identify the type of measurement: length, volume, or weight. To check your answers, see page 63.

1. centimeter
2. kilometer
3. kilogram
4. milliliter
5. microgram

Metric measurement devices

The three basic units in the metric system—the meter, liter, and gram—must be measured with different devices. A meterstick, which resembles a yardstick, is used to measure length. A metric graduate can be used to measure volume in liters. A set of metric weights can be used to measure weight in grams. An enclosed chamber, such as the cylinder formed by the barrel of a syringe, is required to measure a volume of gas.

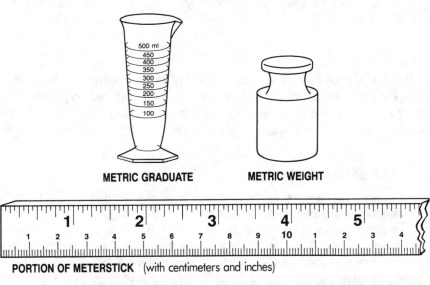

METRIC GRADUATE **METRIC WEIGHT**

PORTION OF METERSTICK (with centimeters and inches)

Metric terms

Besides the three basic units of measurement, the metric system includes other units that are multiples of the basic units. Each of these units has a prefix indicating its relationship to the basic unit and an abbreviation for ease of notation. For example, the most common submultiple of the gram is the *milli*gram (mg), which represents 1/1,000th or 0.001 of a gram. The most common multiple of the gram is the *kilo*gram (kg), which is 1,000 times greater than the gram. These prefixes and others apply to meters, liters, and grams and can be used to express units of measure ranging from kilometers (km) to nanograms (ng) to deciliters (dl). (See *Metric system prefixes, abbreviations, and values* for a listing.)

Metric system prefixes, abbreviations, and values

In the metric system, the addition of a prefix to one of the basic units of measure indicates a multiple or subdivision of that unit. To abbreviate these units of measure, place the prefix abbreviation before the abbreviation g (for gram), l or L (for liter), or m (for meter) For example, abbreviate kilogram as kg and milliliter as ml.

PREFIX	ABBREVIATION	MULTIPLES AND SUBDIVISIONS (FRACTIONS)
kilo	k	1,000
hecto	h	100
deka	dk	10
deci	d	0.1 (1/10th)
centi	c	0.01 (1/100th)
milli	m	0.001 (1/1,000th)
micro	mc	0.000001 (1/1,000,000th)
nano	n	0.000000001 (1/1,000,000,000th)

The metric system also includes one unusual unit of volume, the cubic centimeter (cc). Because the cubic centimeter occupies the same space as one milliliter of liquid, these two units of volume are considered equal and may be used interchangeably. However, cubic centimeters usually are used to refer to gas volume, and milliliters usually are reserved for expressing measurements of liquid volume.

◆ **PRACTICE PROBLEMS**

Metric terms

Identify the unit of measure represented by the following abbreviations. To check your answers, see page 63.

1. mcg
2. ml
3. kg
4. cm
5. L
6. mg

International System of Units

The International Bureau of Weights and Measures adopted the International System of Units (Systeme Internationale or SI) in 1960 to promote standard use of metric abbreviations and prevent mistakes in transcription. Unfortunately, some physicians still may use old abbreviations, which can cause confusion and lead to drug administration errors. Such abbreviations include l (instead of L) to represent liters and gm or GM (instead of g) to represent grams. As additional protection against confusion, some clinicians use L in all liter-related abbreviations, such as mL and dL. However, this is not required and will not be used in this book.

Besides using the recommended abbreviations, remember these general rules when using the metric system.
♦ Always write the numbers that represent quantity *before* the abbreviation.
Examples: 2 kg, 2.5 mg, 37 dl
♦ Always use decimal fractions to represent a part of a whole.
Examples: 3.5 mg, 2.75 ml, 45.656 kg
♦ Always place a zero before the decimal point for amounts that are less than 1. This gives
   special notice to the decimal point.
Examples: 0.8 mg, 0.5 ml, 0.95 mcg
♦ Eliminate extra zeros so that they are not misread.
Examples: 1 mg (not 1.0 mg), 0.5 (not 0.500) ml

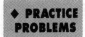

International System of Units

Write out the following metric measurements using the International System of Units. To check your answers, see page 63.

1. four hundred micrograms
2. five-tenths of a milliliter
3. five grams
4. five hundred milligrams
5. two and two-tenths kilograms
6. two-hundredths of a milliliter
7. seven centimeters
8. eight-tenths of a millimeter

Metric conversions

Because the metric system has a decimal basis, conversions between units of measure are relatively easy. To convert a smaller unit to a larger one, move the decimal point to the left or divide by the appropriate multiple. To convert a larger unit to a smaller one, move the decimal point to the right or multiply by the appropriate multiple. (See *Metric conversion scale* for details.) Using the metric conversion scale, the following examples illustrate the process.

Metric conversion scale

When performing metric conversions, you can use the following scale as a guide to decimal placement.

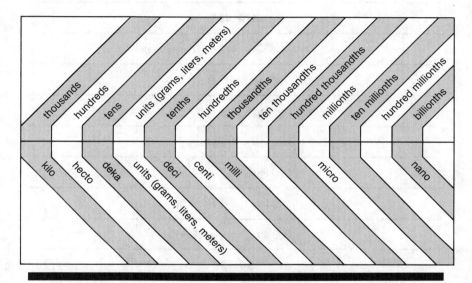

To convert 5 meters (m) to kilometers (km), first count the number of places to the right or left of "meter" to reach "kilo" on the scale. Because a kilometer is three decimal places to the left of a meter (1,000 times larger), move the decimal point to the left, indicating that 5 m equal 0.005 km. Remember to place a zero in front of the decimal point to draw attention to the decimal's presence.

To convert 50 milligrams (mg) to micrograms (mcg), locate "milli" and "micro" on the scale. The Greek symbol μg sometimes is used for microgram but is not recommended in handwriting because it can be misread as mg. Because a microgram is three decimal places to the right of a milligram, or 1,000 times smaller, move the decimal point three places to the right, indicating that 50 mg equal 50,000 mcg.

To convert 250 centiliters (cl) to liters, find these units on the scale. Because a liter is two places to the left of a centiliter, or 100 times larger, move the decimal point two places to the left, indicating that 250 cl equal 2.5 L.

To speed metric conversions, memorize the equivalents of commonly used measures. (See *Metric equivalents,* page 56, for a listing.)

Metric equivalents

This table shows the equivalents of some commonly used metric measures. Several less commonly used measures, such as the hectogram, also are included.

LIQUIDS

1 milliliter	= 1 cubic centimeter
1,000 milliliters	= 1 liter
100 centiliters	= 1 liter
10 deciliters	= 1 liter
10 liters	= 1 dekaliter
100 liters	= 1 hectoliter
1,000 liters	= 1 kiloliter

SOLIDS

1,000 micrograms	= 1 milligram
1,000 milligrams	= 1 gram
100 centigrams	= 1 gram
10 decigrams	= 1 gram
10 grams	= 1 dekagram
100 grams	= 1 hectogram
1,000 grams	= 1 kilogram

Patient situations

An infant weighs 5.2 kg. What is the infant's weight in grams?

◆ Knowing that 1 kg is equal to 1,000 g, set up the following equation:

$$X \text{ g} = 5.2 \text{ kg} \times 1,000 \text{ g/kg}$$
$$X = 5,200 \text{ g}$$

The infant weighs 5,200 g.

A patient received 0.252 L of intravenous (I.V.) fluid. How many milliliters did the patient receive?

◆ Find "liter" and then "milli" on the metric conversion scale. Because "milli" is located three places to the right of "liter," move the decimal point three places to the right, indicating that 0.25 L is equal to 250 ml.

The patient received 250 ml.

The nurse administered 2 g of a medication. How many milligrams of medication did the patient receive?

◆ Knowing that 1 g is equal to 1,000 mg, set up the following equation:

$$X \text{ mg} = 2 \text{ g} \times 1,000 \text{ mg/g}$$
$$X = 2,000 \text{ mg}$$

The patient received 2,000 mg.

During surgery, a patient received 6,500 ml of I.V. fluid. How many liters of fluid did the patient receive?

Find "milli" and then "liter" on the metric conversion scale. Because "liter" is located three places to the left of "milli," move the decimal point three places to the left, indicating that 6,500 ml is equal to 6.5 L.

The patient received 6.5 L of I.V. fluid during surgery.

Metric conversions

Make the following conversions in the metric system. To check your answers, see page 63.

1. 1,800 ml = _____ L
2. 4,250 ml = _____ L
3. 374 mcl = _____ ml
4. 350 ml = _____ L
5. 10 cc = _____ ml
6. 1 L = _____ ml
7. 1 ml = _____ L
8. 58.5 L = _____ ml
9. 220 ml = _____ L
10. 1 mg = _____ mcg
11. 15 g = _____ mg
12. 0.3 L = _____ ml
13. 1 L = _____ dl
14. 95 ml = _____ cc

15. 1 kg = _____ g

16. 1 g = _____ mcg

17. 1 g = _____ mg

18. 52 g = _____ kg

19. 6.2 g = _____ kg

20. 732 g = _____ kg

Metric mathematics

Once you can convert from one metric unit to another, you can solve basic arithmetic problems in metric units. To add, subtract, multiply, or divide different metric units, first convert all quantities to the same metric unit. Unless the problem calls for an answer in a particular unit, use whichever common unit is easiest for you. Then perform the arithmetic operation, as shown in the following examples.

Add 1 kg + 250 mg + 7.5 g, expressing the total in grams.

◆ Convert all units to grams and add.

$$
\begin{array}{rl}
1 \text{ kg} = & 1{,}000.0 \text{ g} \\
250 \text{ mg} = & 0.250 \text{ g} \\
7.5 \text{ g} = + & \underline{7.5 \text{ g}} \\
\text{total} = & 1{,}007.75 \text{ g}
\end{array}
$$

Subtract 3.5 mg from 0.385 g, expressing the answer in micrograms.

◆ Convert all units to micrograms and subtract.

$$
\begin{array}{rl}
0.385 \text{ g} = & 385{,}000 \text{ mcg} \\
3.5 \text{ mg} = - & \underline{3{,}500 \text{ mcg}} \\
\text{answer} = & 381{,}500 \text{ mcg}
\end{array}
$$

Patient situations

A patient received 200 ml from a liter bag of I.V. fluid over the first shift, 375 ml over the second shift, and 175 ml over the third shift. How many milliliters of fluid remain in the I.V. bag?

◆ Determine how much fluid the patient received. To do this, add:

$$
\begin{array}{r}
200 \text{ ml} \\
375 \text{ ml} \\
+ \underline{175 \text{ ml}} \\
750 \text{ ml}
\end{array}
$$

The patient received 750 ml of fluid.

◆ Next, convert all of the measures to the same units. Either 1 L must be converted to milliliters, or 750 ml must be converted to liters. Because the number of milliliters remaining needs to be determined, it will be simpler to convert 1 L to milliliters. 1 L = 1,000 ml.

◆ Compute the amount of fluid remaining by subtracting:

$$
\begin{array}{r}
1{,}000 \text{ ml} \\
- \underline{750 \text{ ml}} \\
250 \text{ ml}
\end{array}
$$

There should be 250 ml of fluid remaining in the patient's I.V. bag.

A patient is to receive 4 g of neomycin before intestinal surgery. Neomycin is available in 500-mg tablets. How many tablets should be administered?

♦ Convert all the measures to the same units. Because the tablets are available in milligrams, convert 4 g to milligrams. On the metric equivalents chart, 1 g is equal to 1,000 mg.

♦ To find how many milligrams are in 4 g, set up a proportion using fractions.

$$\frac{1,000 \text{ mg}}{1 \text{ g}} = \frac{X \text{ mg}}{4 \text{ g}}$$

♦ Solve for X.

$$1 \text{ g} \times X \text{ mg} = 1,000 \text{ mg} \times 4 \text{ g}$$

$$X \text{ mg} = \frac{4,000 \text{ g}}{1 \text{ g}}$$

$$X = 4,000 \text{ mg}$$

♦ Next, determine the number of 500-mg tablets that need to be administered to provide 4,000 mg. Set up a proportion using fractions.

$$\frac{500 \text{ mg}}{1 \text{ tab}} = \frac{4,000 \text{ mg}}{X \text{ tab}}$$

♦ Solve for X.

$$500 \text{ mg} \times X \text{ tab} = 4,000 \text{ mg} \times 1 \text{ tab}$$

$$500 \text{ X} = 4,000$$

$$X = \frac{4,000}{500}$$

$$X = 8 \text{ tablets}$$

The patient should receive 8 tablets of 500 mg each for a dose of 4,000 mg.

A patient must receive 3.5 L of I.V. fluid over 24 hours. Each bag of I.V. fluid contains 500 ml. How many bags of fluid should this patient receive daily?

♦ First, convert the measures to the same units. Because the I.V. fluid is supplied in milliliters, convert 3.5 L to milliliters. (Converting to milliliters also avoids working with decimal fractions, which can become confusing.) Based on the metric conversion scale, 3.5 L = 3,500 ml.

♦ Next, determine the number of 500-ml bags needed to provide 3,500 ml of fluid. To do this, set up a proportion with fractions.

$$500 \text{ ml} = 3,500 \text{ ml}$$

$$1 \text{ bag} = X \text{ bags}$$

♦ Solve for X.

$$500 \text{ ml} \times X \text{ bags} = 3,500 \text{ ml} \times 1 \text{ bag}$$

$$500 \text{ X} = 3,500$$

$$X = \frac{3,500}{500}$$

$$X = 7$$

The patient should receive 7 bags of I.V. fluid over 24 hours.

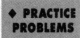
◆ PRACTICE PROBLEMS

Metric mathematics

Calculate the solutions to the following metric problems. To check your answers, see page 64.

1. Add the following and express the total in milligrams:

$$5 \text{ g} + 250 \text{ mg} + 1,600 \text{ mcg.}$$

2. Add the following and express the total in liters:

$$60 \text{ ml} + 0.5 \text{ L} + 600 \text{ ml.}$$

3. Subtract the following and express the answer in milliliters:

$$6 \text{ L} - 500 \text{ ml} - 250 \text{ ml.}$$

4. Subtract the following and express the answer in grams:

$$4 \text{ kg} - 200 \text{ g} - 100 \text{ mg.}$$

5. If one acetaminophen tablet contains 325 mg, half of a tablet should contain how many milligrams?

6. If a patient receives 300 ml of I.V. fluid from a 1-liter bag, how many milliliters remain in the bag? If the patient receives another 250 ml from the same bag, how many milliliters remain in the bag?

7. If the doctor prescribes furosemide (Lasix), 80 mg I.V., and if each furosemide vial contains 20 mg, how many vials would you need to administer the prescribed dose?

8. A patient has received two I.V. antibiotics in 10 ml of fluid each, one antibiotic in 250 ml of fluid, 1 liter of blood, and 800 ml of I.V. fluid. What is this patient's total fluid intake in milliliters?

9. If the nurse divides 4.8 g of a drug into 6 equal doses, how many milligrams will each dose weigh?

10. If the nurse removes 0.5 g, 65 mg, and 4,000 mcg from a vial, how many milligrams have been removed?

11. If the nurse removes 0.5 L, 250 ml, 2.5 L, and 750 ml from a 5-liter bottle, how many milliliters remain?

Review problems

Answer the following questions related to the metric system. To check your answers, see pages 64 and 65.

1. The measurement system based on grams, meters, and liters is the

_____ system.

2. Of the following units of measure, _____, _____, _____,

and _____ belong to the metric system.

ounce	milliliter	scruple
gram	inch	liter
teaspoon	centimeter	dram

3. In the metric system, the basic unit of length is the _____ .

4. In the metric system, the gram is the basic unit used to measure _____ .

5. In the metric system, the basic unit used to measure volume is the _____ .

6. The abbreviation for gram is _____ .

7. The abbreviation for liter is _____ .

8. The abbreviation for microgram is _____ .

9. The abbreviation for milliliter is _____ .

10. The abbreviation for cubic centimeter is _____ .

11. The millimeter equals _____ of a meter.

12. To convert milligrams to grams, move the decimal point _____ places to the

_____ .

13. To convert grams to milligrams, move the decimal point _____ places to the

_____ .

14. To convert kilograms to micrograms, move the decimal point _____ places to the right.

15. 17 g = _____ mg

16. 0.17 g = _____ mg

17. 0.47 g = _____ mg

18. 286 g = _____ mg

19. 160 mcg = _____ mg

20. 1,970 mcg = _____ mg

21. 119,200 mcg = _____ mg

22. 600 mg = _____ g

23. 50,000 mcg = _____ g

24. 125 mcg = _____ mg

25. 3,270 mcg = _____ mg

26. 481,000 mcg = _____ g

27. 305 g = _____ kg

28. 1 mg = _____ mcg

29. 1 mg = _____ ng

30. 0.08 mcg = _____ ng

31. 5.5 g = _____ mg

32. 1 g = _____ ng

33. 33 kg = _____ g

34. 520 mg = _____ g

35. 0.732 g = _____ mcg

36. 0.47 g = _____ mg

37. 25 mcg = _____ mg

38. 0.083 mg = _____ mcg

39. 300 ng = _____ mg

40. 50 mg = _____ mcg

41. Add or subtract the following, expressing the answer in grams.

   a) 0.6 kg + 213 g + 360 mg + 12.4 g

   b) 2 g − 300 mg

   c) 4 kg + 44 g + 344 mg

   d) 1,940 mg − 0.43 g

42. Add or subtract the following, expressing the answer in milliliters.

   a) 210 ml + 0.35 L + 65 cc + 2.6 L

   b) 1 L − 350 ml

43. Add or subtract the following, expressing the answer in milligrams.

   a) 1.4 g + 0.45 g + 180 mcg + 0.24 mg

   b) 30 mg + 30 g + 215 mg + 2 kg + 454 g + 3,000 mg

   c) 0.25 g + 114 mg + 5,000 mcg + 0.03 kg

44. Express the answer to this subtraction problem in micrograms: 25 mg − 144 mcg.

45. Express the answer to this multiplication problem in milligrams: (0.05 g + 0.4 g) × ⅓.

46. If 20 mg, 235 mg, 0.855 g, and 35.5 mg of drug have been removed from a container, how many grams of drug have been removed?

47. How many liters of drug will remain in a 4-L container after 0.5 L and 500 ml have been removed?

48. How many milliliters of drug will be left in a 2-L bottle if 320 ml, 15 ml, 130 ml, and 1.2 L are removed?

49. How many milligrams will each dose weigh if 3.2 g of drug is divided into eight equal doses?

50. Fifteen tablets of an investigational drug weigh 0.825 g. How many milligrams are in each tablet?

51. If 250 mg of cefazolin sodium (Ancef) are administered from a 1-g vial, how many milligrams remain?

52. One phenobarbital (Luminal) tablet weighs 65 mg. How many milligrams do 12 tablets weigh?

53. If a scored digoxin (Lanoxin) tablet contains 0.25 mg of the drug, how many milligrams of the drug would half of the tablet contain?

54. A patient received three different I.V. drugs, each mixed in 50 ml of fluid, over 8 hours. The patient also received 700 ml of I.V. fluid during that time. What was the patient's total I.V. intake in milliliters?

Answers to practice problems

◆ **Units of measurement**

1. length
2. length
3. weight
4. volume
5. weight

◆ *Metric terms*

1. microgram
2. milliliter
3. kilogram
4. centimeter
5. liter
6. milligram

◆ *International System of Units*

1. 400 mcg
2. 0.5 ml
3. 5 g
4. 500 mg
5. 2.2 kg
6. 0.02 ml
7. 7 cm
8. 0.8 mm

◆ *Metric conversions*

1. 1.8 L
2. 4.25 L
3. 0.374 ml
4. 0.35 L
5. 10 ml
6. 1,000 ml
7. 0.001 L
8. 58,500 ml
9. 0.22 L
10. 1,000 mcg
11. 15,000 mg
12. 300 ml
13. 10 dl
14. 95 cc
15. 1,000 g
16. 1,000,000 mcg
17. 1,000 mg
18. 0.052 kg
19. 0.0062 kg
20. 0.732 kg

◆ *Metric mathematics*

1. 5,251.6 mg
2. 1.16 L
3. 5,250 ml
4. 3,799.9 mg
5. 162.5 mg
6. 700 ml, 450 ml
7. 4 vials
8. 2,070 ml
9. 800 mg
10. 569 mg
11. 1,000 ml

Answers to review problems

1. metric
2. gram, milliliter, centimeter, liter
3. meter
4. weight
5. liter
6. g
7. L
8. mcg
9. ml
10. cc
11. $\frac{1}{1,000}$
12. three, left
13. three, right
14. nine
15. 17,000 mg
16. 170 mg
17. 470 mg
18. 286,000 mg
19. 0.16 mg
20. 1.97 mg
21. 119.2 mg
22. 0.6 g

23. 0.05 g

24. 0.125 mg

25. 3.27 mg

26. 0.481 g

27. 0.305 kg

28. 1,000 mcg

29. 1,000,000 ng

30. 80 ng

31. 5,500 mg

32. 1,000,000,000 ng

33. 33,000 g

34. 0.52 g

35. 732,000 mcg

36. 470 mg

37. 0.025 mg

38. 83 mcg

39. 0.0003 mg

40. 50,000 mcg

41. a) 825.76 g

    b) 1.7 g

    c) 4,044.344 g

    d) 1.51 g

42. a) 3,225 ml

    b) 650 ml

43. a) 1,850.42 mg

    b) 2,487,245 mg

    c) 30,369 mg

44. 24,856 mcg

45. 150 mg

46. 1.1455 = 1.146 g

47. 3 L

48. 335 ml

49. 400 mg

50. 55 mg

51. 750 mg

52. 780 mg

53. 0.125 mg

54. 850 ml

Chapter

7

Other Measurement Systems

Although the metric system is the most widely used measurement system in clinical settings, you may use several others, including the apothecaries', household, avoirdupois, unit, and milliequivalent systems. You may use these systems during various drug administration tasks. For example, you may see the apothecaries' system written on a drug order, teach a patient to use a measuring device calibrated in the household system, or use the avoirdupois system to calculate an individualized dosage based on the patient's weight. So to be fully prepared for all drug-related responsibilities, you must be familiar with all of these measurement systems.

Apothecaries' system

Doctors and pharmacists used the apothecaries' system of measurement before the metric system. After the metric system was introduced, however, use of the older system began to decline. Although the apothecaries' system has been phased out and pharmacists may not dispense drugs measured in this system, the nurse may need to check the pharmacist's prescription conversion to the metric system.

Units of measurement

Unlike the metric system, which measures length, volume, and weight, the apothecaries' system measures only volume and weight. In this system, the basic unit for measuring liquid volume is the minim (℞ or m), and the basic unit for measuring solid weight is the grain (gr). To visualize these standards, remember that a minim is about the size of a drop of water, which weighs about the same as 1 grain of wheat. The following mathematical statement sums up this relationship:

$$1 \text{ drop} \approx 1 \text{ minim (℞)} \approx 1 \text{ grain (gr)}.$$

Other units of measure in the apothecaries' system build on these basic units. (See *Apothecaries' measures* for a complete listing.) Many of these units also are used as common household measures. A discussion of the relationship between apothecaries', household, and metric measures appears later in this chapter.

Review of Roman numerals

The apothecaries' system traditionally uses Roman numerals and puts the unit of measurement before the Roman numerals. For example, *5 grains* would be written *grains v*. (Some prescribers

Apothecaries' measures

This table displays the relationships between measures of liquid volume and solid weight in the apothecaries' system.

LIQUID VOLUME
60 minims (♍) = 1 fluidram (f ℨ)
8 f ℨ = 1 fluidounce (f ℥)
16 f ℥ = 1 pint (pt)
2 pt = 1 quart (qt)
4 qt = 1 gallon (gal)
SOLID WEIGHT
60 grains (gr) = 1 dram (ℨ)
8 ℨ = 1 ℥
12 ℥ = 1 pound (lb)

do not follow this traditional convention. Instead, they express apothecaries' system dosages in Arabic numbers followed by units of measurement, such as *5 grains*.)

When used as Roman numerals, the following eight symbols indicate these numeric values:

$$ss = \frac{1}{2} \qquad L = 50$$
$$I = 1 \qquad C = 100$$
$$V = 5 \qquad D = 500$$
$$X = 10 \qquad M = 1{,}000$$

When used in pharmacologic applications, Roman numerals ss (an abbreviation of the Latin word *semis,* meaning half) through X usually are written in lower case. Fractions of less than ½ are written as common fractions using Arabic numbers. Other quantities are expressed by combining letters according to two general rules:

• When a smaller numeral precedes a larger numeral, subtract the smaller numeral. For example,
$$IX = 10 - 1 = 9$$

• When a smaller numeral follows a larger numeral, add the numerals. For example,
$$XI = 10 + 1 = 11$$

To write an Arabic number in Roman numerals, first break the Arabic number into its component parts; then translate the parts into Roman numerals. For example,
$$36 = 30 + 6 = XXXVI$$

Apothecaries' system

Solve the following problems related to the apothecaries' system. To check your answers, see page 76.

Use *Apothecaries' measures,* page 67, to solve the following problems:

1. How many fluidrams make up 1 fluidounce?

2. A prescription calls for 120 grains of a medication. How many drams of the medication is this?

3. Which apothecaries' measure represents the volume of 1 drop of water?

4. A patient must drink 1 quart of water after a diagnostic test. How many pints of water should the patient consume?

Write the following Arabic numbers as Roman numerals:

5. 17

6. 490

Write the following Roman numerals as Arabic numbers:

7. iv

8. XXIX

Household system

Many of the units of liquid measure in the apothecaries' system are identical to those used in the household system of measurement. Because all droppers, teaspoons, tablespoons, and glasses are not alike, however, the household system of liquid measurement can be used for approximate measures only. You shouldn't use the household system to measure medications, but the patient might use it. You should use the metric system.

Most liquid medications are prescribed and dispensed in the metric system. To ensure the accuracy of dosages measured in the household system, teach the patient to measure the prescribed dosage using household measures. (See *Household measures.*) Also suggest devices for more accurate drug measurement. (See *Teaching about liquid measurement devices,* page 70.)

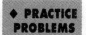

Household system

Perform the following conversions in the household system. To check your answers, see page 76.

1. 3 tsp = _____ Tbs

2. 1 tsp = _____ gtt

3. 6 Tbs = _____ oz

4. 1 pt = _____ Tbs

5. 1 pt and 8 oz = _____ cups

Avoirdupois system

The nurse should be aware of the avoirdupois system because it is used for ordering and purchasing some pharmaceutical products and for weighing patients in some clinical settings.

In the avoirdupois system, the solid measures or units of weight include grains (gr), ounces (437.5 gr), and pounds (16 oz or 7,000 gr). Note that the apothecaries' pound equals 12 oz, but the avoirdupois pound equals 16 oz.

Household measures

This table shows the equivalents of the most commonly used household measures, which are used to measure liquid volume. Note: The abbreviations "t" (teaspoon) and "T" (tablespoon) should be avoided because they carry a high potential for error when written quickly. Always clarify a prescription that includes these symbols.

LIQUIDS

60 drops (gtt) = 1 teaspoon (tsp)
3 tsp = 1 tablespoon (Tbs)
2 Tbs = 1 ounce (oz)
8 oz = 1 cup
16 oz (2 cups) = 1 pint (pt)
2 pt = 1 quart (qt)
4 qt = 1 gallon (gal)

◆ PRACTICE PROBLEMS

Avoirdupois system

Perform the following conversions in the avoirdupois system. To check your answers, see page 76.

1. 1 lb = _____ oz
2. 1 lb = _____ gr
3. 7,000 gr = _____ oz
4. 1 oz = _____ gr

Unit system

Some drugs are measured in units, such as United States Pharmacopeia (USP) units or International Units (IU). The most common drug measured in units (U) is insulin, which comes in 10-ml multidose vials of U-40 or U-100 strength. With this drug, the U refers to the number of units of insulin per milliliter. For example, 1 ml of U-40 insulin contains 40 units; 1 ml of U-100 insulin contains 100 units. Use of U-40 insulin has declined in recent years; the U-100 strength, which is based on metric measurement, makes measurement in a standard syringe easier. (For more information, see Chapter 16, Insulin Dosage Calculation.)

Other drugs also are measured in units. For example, the anticoagulant heparin is available in liquid forms that contain 10 to 20,000 U/ml for parenteral use. Bacitracin, an antibiotic, is available in a topical form that contains 50 U/ml. Penicillins G and V are available in different

Teaching about liquid measurement devices

The nurse should teach the patient how to use several devices that will help ensure accurate dosage measurements.

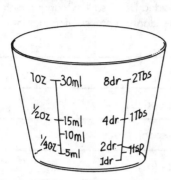

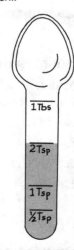

MEDICATION CUP
(calibrated in household, metric, and apothecaries' systems)

Teach the patient to set the cup on a counter and check the fluid measurement at eye level.

DROPPER
(calibrated in household or metric systems or in terms of medication strength or concentration)

Teach the patient to hold the dropper at eye level to check the fluid measurement.

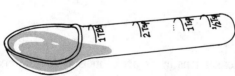
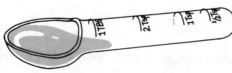

HOLLOW-HANDLE SPOON
(calibrated in teaspoons and tablespoons)
Teach the patient to check the dose after filling by holding the spoon upright at eye level. To administer, the patient tilts the spoon until the medication fills the bowl of the spoon and then places the spoon in the mouth.

forms that contain 400,000 U/ml (approximately equal to 250 mg) or 800,000 U/ml (approximately equal to 500 mg). The hormone calcitonin is measured in IU, as are the fat-soluble vitamins A, D, and E. Some forms of vitamins A and D also are measured in USP units.

To calculate the dose to be administered when the medication is available in units, use the following proportion:

$$\frac{\text{amount of drug (ml)}}{\text{dose of drug required (U)}} = \frac{1 \text{ ml}}{\text{drug available (U)}}$$

Patient situation

A patient requires 16 U of insulin daily. How many milliliters of U-100 insulin should be given?

♦ Set up the proportion.

$$\frac{X \text{ ml}}{16 \text{ U}} = \frac{1 \text{ ml}}{100 \text{ U}}$$

♦ Solve for X.

$$X \text{ ml} \times 100 \text{ U} = 16 \text{ U} \times 1 \text{ ml}$$

$$X = \frac{16 \text{ ml}}{100}$$

$$X = 0.16 \text{ ml}$$

The patient should be given 0.16 ml of insulin.

Unit system

Solve the following problems in the unit system. To check your answers, see page 76.

1. You must add 25,000 U of heparin to 250 ml of I.V. fluid. Heparin is supplied in 5,000 U/ml of fluid. How many milliliters of heparin should you add to the I.V. fluid?

2. A patient takes 5 U of regular insulin (U-100) and 15 U of NPH insulin (U-100) every morning. How many milliliters of insulin does the patient take each day?

3. The doctor prescribes 200,000 U of penicillin G for a patient. Because the pharmacy has no vials that contain 200,000 U/ml, it provides a vial labelled penicillin G 800,000 U/ml. How many milliliters should you administer?

4. A hospitalized patient requires 45 U of NPH insulin (U-100) every morning. How many milliliters of insulin should you administer?

Milliequivalent system

Electrolytes are measured in milliequivalents (mEq). Drug manufacturers provide information about the number of metric units required to provide the prescribed number of milliequivalents. For example, the manufacturer's instructions may indicate that 1 ml equals 4 mEq.

A doctor usually orders the electrolyte potassium chloride in milliequivalents. Potassium preparations for I.V., oral, or other use are available as liquid (elixir and parenteral) and solid (powder and tablet) forms.

Patient situations

A patient who is receiving medications and feedings through a nasogastric tube is to receive 10 mEq of potassium chloride. The label on the container of elixir states **Potassium Chloride, 30 mEq = 30 ml.** *How many milliliters must be given to the patient?*

◆ Set up the proportion.

$$\frac{X \text{ ml}}{10 \text{ mEq}} = \frac{30 \text{ ml}}{30 \text{ mEq}}$$

◆ Solve for X.

$$X \text{ ml} \times 30 \text{ mEq} = 10 \text{ mEq} \times 30 \text{ ml}$$

$$X = \frac{300 \text{ ml}}{30}$$

$$X = 10 \text{ ml}$$

More simply, if a solution contains 30 mEq in 30 ml, it contains 1 mEq/ml. Thus, if 10 mEq is needed, 10 ml should be given to the patient.

A patient needs 20 mEq of potassium chloride added to 1 L of I.V. fluids. The available vial of potassium chloride contains 2 mEq/ml. How many milliliters of potassium chloride must be added to the I.V. fluid?

◆ Set up the ratio.

$$2 \text{ mEq} : 1 \text{ ml} :: 20 \text{ mEq} : X \text{ ml}$$

◆ Solve for X.

$$2 \text{ mEq} \times X \text{ ml} = 1 \text{ ml} \times 20 \text{ mEq}$$

$$X \text{ ml} = \frac{20}{2}$$

$$X = 10 \text{ ml}$$

Ten milliliters of potassium chloride should be added to the I.V. fluid.

Milliequivalent system

Solve the following problems in the milliequivalent system. To check your answers, see page 76.

1. A patient must receive 25 mEq of sodium bicarbonate. The vial from the pharmacy contains 50 mEq in every 50 ml. How many milliliters of the solution should you administer?

2. You need to prepare a 30-mEq dose of potassium chloride from a vial labeled 40 mEq of potassium chloride per 20 ml. How many milliliters should you prepare?

3. The doctor prescribes 30 mEq of potassium chloride oral solution for a patient. The solution provides 20 mEq in every 15 ml. How many milliliters of solution should the patient receive?

Equivalent measures among systems

In clinical practice, a doctor's order for medication may be written in one system of measurement, and the medication may be available in a different system. For example, the doctor may order a medication in grains, and the medication may be available in milligrams. To convert medication orders from one system to another, the nurse must know the equivalent measures among systems of measurement.

Although references and charts that list equivalent measures among systems usually are available in the clinical setting, most nurses memorize the most frequently used equivalents. (See *Equivalent measures* for a list of common equivalents among the metric, apothecaries', and household systems.)

Equivalent measures

The following table shows some *approximate* liquid equivalents among the household, apothecaries', and metric systems.

An agency or institution may acknowledge a particular set of equivalents as its official standard for exchange among systems. All health care professionals prescribing, dispensing, or administering drugs under such an agency's purview should abide by the established protocol. If no protocol exists, use the equivalent that is easiest to manipulate in any given computation problem.

HOUSEHOLD	APOTHECARIES'	METRIC
1 drop (gtt)	1 minim (♏)	0.06 milliliter (ml)
15 or 16 gtt	15 or 16 ♏	1 ml
1 teaspoon (tsp)	1 fluidram (f₃)	4 or 5 ml
1 tablespoon (Tbs)	½ fluidounce (f ℥)	15 or 16 ml
2 Tbs	1 f ℥	30 or 32 ml
1 cup	8 f ℥	240 or 250 ml
1 pint (pt)	16 f ℥	473, 480, or 500 ml
1 quart (qt)	32 f ℥	946, 960, or 1,000 ml (1 liter)
1 gallon (gal)	128 f ℥	3,785, 3,840, or 4,000 ml

The following table shows some *approximate* solid equivalents among the avoirdupois, apothecaries', and metric systems.

AVOIRDUPOIS	APOTHECARIES'	METRIC
1 grain (gr)	1 grain (gr)	0.06 or 0.065 gram (g)
15.4 gr	15 gr	1 g
1 ounce	480 gr	28.35 g
1 pound (lb)	1.33 pounds (lb)	454 g
2.2 lb	2.7 lb	1 kg

The plastic medication cup used for liquid preparations also is readily available in the clinical area, providing a quick reference for equivalents among measures in the metric, apothecaries', and household systems. Additionally, some syringes are labeled in the metric and apothecaries' systems and can be used as a quick reference for liquid measures between these two systems.

Patient situation

A patient has been taking 15 ml of a medication while hospitalized and is to continue taking this dose at home. The patient's medication cup at home is marked in ounces. How many ounces per dose should the patient take at home?

◆ Set up a proportion. Because 30 ml is equivalent to 1 oz, the proportion would be:

$$\frac{30 \text{ ml}}{1 \text{ oz}} = \frac{15 \text{ ml}}{X \text{ oz}}$$

$$30 X = 1 \times 15$$

$$X = \frac{15}{30}$$

$$X = \frac{1}{2} \text{ oz}$$

◆ Teach the patient how much medication to take using a plastic medication cup labeled in milliliters and ounces.

◆ PRACTICE PROBLEMS

Equivalent measures among systems

Solve the following problems about equivalent measures. To check your answers, see page 76.

1. A patient must restrict daily fluid intake to 360 ml. Upon returning home, the patient can consume a maximum of how many cups of fluid a day?

2. The doctor prescribes 10 gr of a medication for a patient. How many milligrams of medication should the patient receive?

3. A patient must take 1 tsp of a medication. How many milliliters of medication is this?

4. A patient must take 2 Tbs of a medication. How many milliliters of medication is this?

Review problems

Solve the following problems related to various measurement systems. To check your answers, see page 77.

Answer the following questions about the apothecaries' system:

1. What apothecaries' measure represents the volume of 1 drop of water?

2. What is the abbreviation for 4½ fluidrams as it appears in prescriptions?

3. What is the abbreviation for 12 fluidounces as it appears in prescriptions?

4. ʒ i = gr _____

5. gr CCX = ʒ _____

6. f ʒ iv = f ℥ _____

Write the following Arabic numbers as Roman numerals:

7. 15

8. 110

Write the following Roman numerals as Arabic numbers:

9. viii

10. XLVI

Perform the following conversions in the household system:

11. 3 Tbs = _____ tsp

12. ½ cup = _____ Tbs

13. ½ tsp = _____ gtt

14. 1 Tbs = _____ gtt

Solve these problems in the avoirdupois system:

15. 7 lb = _____ oz

16. 256 oz = _____ lb

17. 3,500 gr = _____ oz

18. 1.5 lb = _____ gr

Solve these problems in the unit system:

19. A patient must receive 36 U of NPH insulin (U-100). How many milliliters of insulin is this?

20. The doctor orders 5,000 U of heparin S.C. As supplied, the heparin contains 5,000 U in 0.5 ml of fluid. How many milliliters of heparin should the patient receive?

21. A patient needs a dose of 35 U of NPH (U-100) insulin and 8 U of regular (U-100) insulin. How many milliliters of insulin, in total, should the patient receive?

22. For a patient who must receive 400,000 U of penicillin G, the pharmacy sends a vial that contains 800,000 U/ml. How many milliliters should you administer?

23. How many units are contained in 1 ml of U-40 insulin?

Solve these problems in the milliequivalent system:

24. A patient needs to have 60 mEq of potassium solution added to 1 L of I.V. fluid. The solution contains 2 mEq per 1 ml. How many milliliters should you add?

25. A patient needs to receive 35 mEq of sodium bicarbonate from a vial that contains 50 mEq in 50 ml of solution. How many milliliters should you administer?

26. A vial of calcium gluconate contains 0.465 mEq/ml. If the doctor orders a dose of 2.325 mEq, how many milliliters should you give?

27. If a patient receives 20 ml of potassium chloride in a dosage strength of 2 mEq/ml, how many milliequivalents of the drug should the patient receive?

Answer these questions about equivalent measures:

28. The doctor prescribes 1 fluidram of cough medicine for a child. How many teaspoons is that?

29. A child needs 240 mg of acetaminophen elixir, which is available in a dosage strength of 120 mg/5 ml. How many teaspoons of the drug should the child receive?

30. A patient needs to have an enema that is prepared with 1 L of water. If the patient prepares the enema at home, how many quarts of water should he use?

31. A doctor's order reads *2 Tbs Milk of Magnesia.* How many milliliters is this?

Answers to practice problems

◆ Apothecaries' system

1. 8 fluidrams

2. 2 drams

3. 1 minim

4. 2 pints

5. XVII

6. CDXC

7. 4

8. 29

◆ Household system

1. 1 Tbs

2. 60 gtt

3. 3 oz

4. 32 Tbs

5. 3 cups

◆ Avoirdupois system

1. 16 oz

2. 7,000 gr

3. 16 oz

4. 437.5 gr

◆ Unit system

1. 5 ml

2. 0.2 ml

3. 0.25 ml

4. 0.45 ml

◆ Milliequivalent system

1. 25 ml

2. 15 ml

3. 22.5 ml

◆ Equivalent measures among systems

1. 1½ cups

2. 600 mg

3. 4 or 5 ml

4. 30 or 32 ml

Answers to review problems

1. ℳ i
2. ℥ ivss
3. ℥ XII
4. gr LX
5. ℥ iiiss
6. ℥ XXXII
7. XV
8. CX
9. 8
10. 46
11. 9 tsp
12. 8 Tbs
13. 30 gtt
14. 180 gtt
15. 112 oz
16. 16 lb
17. 8 oz
18. 10,500 gr
19. 0.36 ml
20. 0.5 ml
21. 0.43 ml
22. 0.5 ml
23. 40 U
24. 30 ml
25. 35 ml
26. 5 ml
27. 40 mEq
28. 1 tsp
29. 2 tsp
30. 1 qt
31. 30 ml

UNIT 3

◆

Drug Orders and Medication Records

The safe, accurate administration of patient medications is an essential nursing responsibility. By being aware of pharmacologic terminology and by following medication administration protocols, the nurse can reduce the risk of medication errors.

To help the nurse reach that goal, Unit 3 highlights interpretation of drug orders and documentation of drug administration. Chapter 8 focuses on drug orders. After describing the components of drug orders, it provides an opportunity to interpret orders. It also explains how to handle unclear orders. Chapter 9 introduces medication administration records (MARs) and discusses the importance of accurate documentation when transcribing orders and administering drugs.

The skills described in this unit are extremely important to the nurse. An error in order interpretation, order transcription, or documentation of drug administration could lead to multiple drug administration errors by other nurses who refer to the MAR. Therefore, the nurse must be prepared to handle these responsibilities expertly.

Chapter

Drug Orders

To administer drugs safely to any patient, the nurse must be able to read and interpret drug orders correctly. Chapter 8 helps prepare the nurse for these tasks and outlines the nurse's responsibility in handling drug orders that are unclear.

Understanding drug orders

Before you can read and interpret drug orders, you must understand their uses and components.

In an outpatient setting, a doctor or other health care professional licensed to prescribe medications may write a drug order on a prescription form and give it directly to the patient. In turn, the patient gives the order to a pharmacist, who dispenses the drug to the patient for home use. In a hospital, the prescriber can generate a drug order by:
• entering the order into the computer system, which sends it to the pharmacy and the nurses' station, or
• writing the drug order on the doctor's order sheet in the patient's chart.

Because an order sheet must include complete patient information, it is usually stamped with the patient's admission data plate. Each order also must include all of the following information:
• date and time of the order
• name of drug (generic or proprietary)
• dosage form (in metric, apothecaries', or household measurements)
• route of administration (P.O., I.M., S.C., I.V., P.R., P.V., S.L., or topical; in some agencies, if the route is not given, the oral route may be assumed)
• administration schedule (as times per day or as hour intervals)
• any restrictions or specifications related to the order
• the doctor's signature or, in a computerized system, the doctor's name and code number (either may follow a group of orders)
• the doctor's issued registration number for controlled drugs (if applicable).

If any of this required information is missing, the nurse must question and clarify the order before signing the transcription. A contact copy or carbon copy of the order is sent to the pharmacy, where the drug is dispensed according to facility policy. To limit the risk of error, make sure that only approved abbreviations are used in the order. The actual times at which the drug is administered depend on facility policy (for drugs given a specific number of times per day) and on the drug's nature and onset and duration of action. These actual times are recorded on the medication administration record (MAR); the drug should be administered within ½ hour before or after the times specified.

Agencies have policies regarding how frequently drug orders must be renewed. Narcotics, for example, may need to be reordered every 24, 48, or 72 hours, according to facility policy. This enables health care professionals to reevaluate the patient's need for the medication and to adjust the dosage or frequency of administration, if necessary.

If treatment with a medication must be halted before the original order has run out, the doctor must write a new order to discontinue the drug. Clarity in such an order also is necessary. For example, if a doctor writes *D/C K,* and the patient is receiving vitamin K and potassium chloride (KCl), the nurse must contact the doctor to clarify which medication is to be discontinued.

To avoid medication errors and ensure patient safety, the nurse should double check the order at the patient's bedside. Before administering any medication, consider the five "rights" of drug administration:
- right drug
- right dose
- right route
- right time
- right patient.

◆ **PRACTICE PROBLEMS**

Understanding drug orders

Answer the following questions about drug orders. To check your answers, see page 89.

1. Every drug order must include the _____ of administration as well as other information.

2. In a computerized system, the doctor's name and _____ must accompany each drug order.

3. To avoid drug errors and ensure patient safety, the nurse must _____ _____ the order at the patient's bedside.

4. The five "rights" of drug administration include: the right drug, right dose, right route, right time, and right _____ .

Reading drug orders

To read drug orders, you must be able to interpret abbreviations that are commonly used by doctors. (See *Common pharmacologic abbreviations* for a list.)

Common pharmacologic abbreviations

To transcribe medication orders and document drug administration accurately, review the following commonly used abbreviations for drug measurements, dosage forms, routes and times of administration, and related terms. Remember that abbreviations are subject to misinterpretation, especially if written carelessly or quickly. If an abbreviation seems unusual or does not make sense, *always* question the order, clarify the terms, and clearly *write out* the correct term in the revision and transcription.

DRUG AND SOLUTION MEASUREMENTS

cc	cubic centimeter	mEq	milliequivalent
f ℨ	fluidram	mg	milligram
f ℥ or oz	fluidounce	ml	milliliter
g	gram	♏	minim
gal	gallon	pt	pint
gr	grain	qt	quart
gtt	drop	ss	one-half
kg	kilogram	Tbs	tablespoon
L	liter	tsp	teaspoon
mcg	microgram	U	unit

DRUG DOSAGE FORMS

cap	capsule	sp	spirits
DS	double strength	supp	suppository
elix	elixir	susp	suspension
LA	long-acting	syr	syrup
liq	liquid	tab	tablet
S.A.	sustained action	tinct or tr	tincture
S.R.	sustained release	ung or oint	ointment
sol	solution		

ROUTES OF DRUG ADMINISTRATION

A.D.	right ear	O.S.	left eye
A.S.	left ear	O.D.	right eye
A.U.	each ear	O.U.	each eye

(continued)

Common pharmacologic abbreviations *(continued)*

ROUTES OF DRUG ADMINISTRATION *(continued)*

I.M.	intramuscular	P.O. or p.o.	by mouth
I.T.	intrathecal	puff	by oral inhalation
I.V.	intravenous	R or P.R.	by rectum
IVPB	intravenous piggyback	R	right
L	left	S.C. or SQ	subcutaneous
NGT	nasogastric tube	SL or sl	sublingual
V or P.V.	vaginally	S&S	swish and swallow

TIMES OF DRUG ADMINISTRATION

a.c.	before meals	q.h.	every hour
ad lib	as desired	q2h, q3h, etc.	every 2 hours, every 3 hours, etc.
b.i.d.	twice a day	q.i.d.	four times a day
h.s.	at bedtime	q.n.	every night
p.c.	after meals	q.o.d.	every other day
p.r.n.	as needed	STAT	immediately
q.a.m. or Q.M.	every morning	t.i.d.	three times a day
q.d. or Q.D.	every day		

MISCELLANEOUS ABBREVIATIONS

AMA	against medical advice	Rx	treatment, prescription
ASAP	as soon as possible	$\bar{s}$	without
$\bar{c}$	with	TO	telephone order
D/C or dc	discontinue	VO	verbal order
HO	house officer	≈	approximately equal to
KVO	keep vein open	>	greater than
MR	may repeat	<	less than
NKA	no known allergies	↑	increase
N.P.O.	nothing by mouth	↓	decrease

Keep these guidelines in mind when interpreting drug orders:
• The generic name of a drug should appear in lowercase letters only.
• The trade, or brand, name of a drug should begin with a capital letter.
• Drug abbreviations should be avoided, but when used should appear in all capital letters.
• Drug orders should be written in the following order: drug name, dosage, administration route, and frequency of administration (such as Lasix 40 mg I.V. q12h.)

Review *Interpreting drug orders* for examples of drug orders and their interpretations.

Interpreting drug orders

The following examples illustrate how to read and interpret a wide range of drug orders.

DRUG ORDER	INTERPRETATION
Colace 100 mg P.O. b.i.d. p.c.	Give 100 mg of Colace by mouth twice a day after meals.
Vistaril 25 mg I.M. q3h p.r.n.	Give 25 mg of Vistaril intramuscularly every 3 hours, as needed.
↑ Duramorph to 6 mg I.V. q8h	Increase Duramorph to 6 mg intravenously every 8 hours.
folic acid 1 mg P.O. daily	Give 1 mg of folic acid by mouth daily.
Minipress 4 mg P.O. q6h, hold for sys BP <120	Give 4 mg of Minipress by mouth every 6 hours; withhold drug if the systolic blood pressure falls below 120 mm Hg.
nifedipine 30 mg SL q4h	Give 30 mg of nifedipine sublingually every 4 hours.
Begin ASA 325 mg P.O. daily	Begin giving 325 mg of aspirin by mouth daily.
Persantine 75 mg P.O. t.i.d.	Give 75 mg of Persantine by mouth three times a day.
aspirin gr v P.O. t.i.d.	Give 5 grains of aspirin by mouth three times a day.
Vasotec 2.5 mg P.O. daily	Give 2.5 mg of Vasotec by mouth daily.
1,000 ml D_5W c̄ KCl 20 mEq I.V. at 100 ml/h	Give 1,000 ml of dextrose 5% in water with 20 mEq of potassium chloride intravenously at a rate of 100 ml/hour.
D/C PCN I.V., start PCN-G 800,000 U P.O. q6h	Discontinue I.V. penicillin; start 800,000 units of penicillin G by mouth every 6 hours.
diphenhydramine 25-50 mg P.O. h.s. p.r.n.	Give 25 to 50 mg of diphenhydramine by mouth at bedtime, as needed.

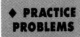

Reading drug orders

Answer the following questions about reading drug orders. To check your answers, see page 89.

Provide the accepted abbreviation for the italicized phrases in the following sentences.

1. Administer a medication *every 4 hours.* _____

2. Administer a medication *as needed.* _____

3. *Discontinue* the I.V. fluids. _____

4. The doctor called with a *telephone order.* _____

5. Administer the following medication *before meals.* _____

Interpret the following drug orders.

6. acetaminophen 650 mg P.R. q4h p.r.n. temperature > 101.5°

_____

_____

7. Coumadin 2.5 mg P.O. daily

_____

_____

8. Narcan 0.4 mg I.V. STAT

_____

_____

9. Pepcid 20 mg I.V. q12h

_____

_____

10. Novolin N insulin 32 U S.C. q.a.m.

_____

_____

11. D/C nifedipine 20 mg P.O. q4h

_____

_____

12. 1 L NSS c̄ KCl 40 mEq I.V. at 250 ml/h

_____

_____

Write the following as drug orders.

13. Increase the nifedipine dose to 20 mg sublingually every 6 hours.

_____

14. Immediately administer 80 mg of Lasix intravenously.

_____

15. Administer 1 mg Dilaudid intravenously every 2 hours.

_____

16. Decrease the intravenous flow rate of 5% dextrose in normal saline to 125 ml per hour.

_____

17. Administer 50 mg of Benadryl by mouth every night at bedtime.

_____

Handling unclear drug orders

The nurse also needs to know how to handle unclear orders. For example, many doctors develop their own abbreviations and notations for drug orders; others have illegible handwriting. (See *Coping with difficult drug orders* for samples.) In either case, the nurse must contact the doctor for clarification. The nurse is responsible for ensuring that the proper drug, strength, and dosage form are transcribed onto the Kardex or MAR and given to the patient.

Coping with difficult drug orders

The combination of poor handwriting and inappropriate abbreviations on a drug order can lead to confusion and medication errors. For any drug order that does not clearly state the drug name, amount, route of administration, and timing of administration, the nurse should contact the doctor. The examples below illustrate drug orders that need clarification.

The nurse also needs to know how to handle orders for drug doses in strengths that are not commercially available. For example, phenytoin is available only in 100-mg capsules or vials. If the doctor orders phenytoin 300 mg P.O. or I.V., the nurse will need to calculate the number of capsules or vials required to provide the correct dose. (Subsequent chapters provide detailed information about dosage calculation methods.)

◆ **PRACTICE PROBLEMS**

Handling unclear drug orders

Fill in the blanks in the following statements about handling unclear drug orders. To check your answers, see page 89.

1. If the doctor writes an illegible drug order, the nurse should contact the doctor for _____ .

2. The nurse must ensure that the proper drug, strength, and _____ form are transcribed onto the Kardex or MAR.

3. If the doctor orders a drug that is not available in the strength ordered, the nurse must perform a dosage _____ to determine the number of capsules or vials needed to provide the correct dose.

Review problems

Answer the following questions about drug orders. To check your answers, see pages 89 and 90.

1. What component is missing from the following drug order?
9/15, 4 P.M., morphine sulfate 4 mg I.V., Dr. Joseph Crane, 37845 _____

2. Each drug order must include the date and time of the _____ .

3. Before administering any drug, the nurse should make sure that the right drug is being given in the right dose by the right route at the right _____ to the right patient.

4. The five "rights" of drug administration were devised to ensure patient _____ .

Interpret the following doctors' orders.

5. Compazine 5 mg I.M. q6h p.r.n. for N/V

_____

_____

6. Nembutal 40 mg P.O. h.s. p.r.n.

_____

_____

7. digoxin 0.25 mg P.O. Q.D., hold for apical pulse < 60

_____

_____

8. lidocaine 50 mg I.V. bolus at 25 mg/min STAT and q8-10 min × 1 p.r.n.

_____

_____

9. regular insulin 10 U I.V. STAT

_____

10. D/C Isuprel I.V. drip

_____

11. Bronkometer inhaler 1 puff q4h p.r.n.

_____

_____

12. nifedipine 20 mg SL q8h

_____

13. hydroxyzine 25 mg I.M. q4h p.r.n. anxiety

_____

14. $FeSO_4$ 325 mg P.O. t.i.d. a.c.

_____

15. Dalmane 30 mg P.O. h.s. p.r.n. MR $\times$ 1

_____

16. Change I.V. from D_5NS to $D_5\frac{1}{2}$ NS

_____

17. Procardia 10 mg P.O. t.i.d. & h.s.

_____

18. oxacillin 1 g IVPB q6h $\times$ 24 hours

_____

_____

19. D_5LR I.V. at 100 ml/h

_____

20. Chloroptic solution 0.5% 2 gtt O.D. q.i.d.

_____

_____

Write the following as drug orders.

21. Administer 60 mg of pseudoephedrine by mouth every 4 to 6 hours, as needed, for congestion.

_____

22. Administer 2 grams of Unipen by piggyback intravenous infusion every 6 hours.

_____

23. Administer 200 mg of phenytoin suspension every morning and 150 mg every night through a nasogastric tube.

_____

24. Change the intravenous infusion to 1,000 ml of 5% dextrose in one-third normal saline delivered at a rate of 125 ml/hour.

_____

25. Administer 500 mg of ampicillin diluted in 50 ml of normal saline solution every 6 hours for four doses; then change to 500 mg by mouth every 6 hours for 10 days; then discontinue.

_____

26. Administer 30 mg of codeine by mouth every 4 hours, as necessary, for pain.

_____

27. Immediately administer 50 mg of Benadryl by mouth.

_____

28. Decrease the intravenous infusion rate of dextrose 5% in water to 100 ml/hour.

_____

29. Administer 1 mg of colchicine every hour for 4 hours; then change to 0.6 mg by mouth three times a day, before meals.

_____

30. Administer 1 mg of Ativan by mouth three times a day; then administer 2 mg at bedtime.

_____

31. Administer 40 mg of Mylicon by mouth after meals, as necessary.

_____

32. Administer 1 tablespoon of Metamucil mixed in 8 ounces of water or juice by mouth daily.

_____

33. Administer 4 ml of Mycostatin suspension (strength: 100,000 units/ml) four times a day, and have patient swish in mouth, then swallow.

_____

34. Administer 40 mg of propranolol by mouth every 8 hours. Hold the dose if the patient's systolic blood pressure falls below 100 mm Hg.

_____

35. Administer 250 mg of Aldomet by mouth every 12 hours (for a total of four doses); then increase the dosage to 500 mg by mouth every 12 hours.

_____

36. For any drug order that does not clearly state the drug name, amount, administration route, and administration schedule, the nurse should contact the _____ .

Answers to practice problems

◆ Understanding drug orders

1. route
2. code number
3. double check
4. patient

◆ Reading drug orders

1. q4h
2. p.r.n.
3. D/C or dc
4. TO
5. a.c.
6. Administer 650 mg of acetaminophen by rectum every 4 hours, as needed for a temperature above 101.5° F.
7. Administer 2.5 mg of Coumadin by mouth daily.
8. Immediately administer 0.4 mg of Narcan intravenously.
9. Administer 20 mg of Pepcid intravenously every 12 hours.
10. Administer 32 units of Novolin N insulin subcutaneously every morning.
11. Discontinue administration of 20 mg of nifedipine by mouth every 4 hours.
12. Administer 1 L of intravenous normal saline solution with 40 mEq of potassium chloride added and run it at 250 ml per hour.
13. ↑ nifedipine to 20 mg SL q6h
14. Lasix 80 mg I.V. STAT
15. Dilaudid 1 mg I.V. q2h
16. ↓ D_5NSS I.V. to 125 ml/h
17. Benadryl 50 mg P.O. h.s.

◆ Handling unclear drug orders

1. clarification
2. dosage
3. calculation

Answers to review problems

1. administration schedule
2. order
3. time
4. safety

5. Administer 5 mg of Compazine by intramuscular injection every 6 hours, as needed, for nausea or vomiting.

6. Administer 40 mg of Nembutal by mouth at bedtime, as needed.

7. Administer 0.25 mg of digoxin by mouth daily; hold for apical pulse rate less than 60 beats/ minute.

8. Immediately administer 50 mg of lidocaine by intravenous bolus infusion at a rate of 25 mg/ minute; if necessary, repeat the dose after 8 to 10 minutes, one time only.

9. Immediately administer 10 U of regular insulin intravenously.

10. Discontinue the intravenous infusion of Isuprel.

11. Administer 1 oral inhalation of Bronkometer every 4 hours, as needed.

12. Administer 20 mg of nifedipine sublingually every 8 hours.

13. Administer 25 mg of hydroxyzine by intramuscular injection every 4 hours, as needed, for anxiety.

14. Administer 325 mg of ferrous sulfate by mouth three times a day before meals.

15. Administer 30 mg of Dalmane by mouth at bedtime, as needed. May repeat once during the night if necessary.

16. Change the patient's intravenous fluid from 5% dextrose in normal saline to 5% dextrose in half-normal saline.

17. Administer 10 mg of Procardia by mouth three times a day and at bedtime.

18. Administer four 1-gram doses of oxacillin by piggyback intravenous infusion, 6 hours apart.

19. Administer 5% dextrose in Ringer's lactate solution by intravenous infusion at a rate of 100 ml/hour.

20. Place 2 drops of 0.5% Chloroptic solution in the right eye four times a day.

21. pseudoephedrine 60 mg P.O. q4-6h p.r.n. congestion

22. Unipen 2 g IVPB q6h

23. phenytoin susp 200 mg per NGT q.a.m. and 150 mg per NGT q.n.

24. Change I.V. to 1,000 ml $D_5$0.33 NS at 125 ml/h.

25. ampicillin 500 mg in 50 ml NSS IVPB q6h × 4 doses, then 500 mg P.O. q6h × 10 days, then D/C

26. codeine 30 mg P.O. q4h p.r.n. pain

27. Benadryl 50 mg P.O. STAT

28. ↓ D_5W I.V. to 100 ml/h

29. colchicine 1 mg P.O. q1h × 4, then 0.6 mg P.O. t.i.d. a.c.

30. Ativan 1 mg P.O. t.i.d. and 2 mg h.s.

31. Mylicon 40 mg P.O. p.c. p.r.n.

32. Metamucil 1 Tbs in 8 oz of water or juice P.O. daily

33. Mycostatin susp (100,000 U/ml) 4 ml q.i.d. S&S

34. propranolol 40 mg P.O. q8h, hold if systolic BP < 100

35. Aldomet 250 mg P.O. q12h × 48h, then ↑ to 500 mg P.O. q12h

36. doctor

Chapter

9

Medication Records

Maintaining accurate medication records is a vital nursing responsibility for legal and patient-safety reasons. In terms of legal concerns, if medication administration wasn't documented, it didn't happen. In terms of patient safety, missed or inaccurate documentation of medication administration can lead to drug errors that can jeopardize the patient's health.

Various types of medication administration record systems are available. For medication charting, some facilities use a Kardex, a set of large index cards in a hinged file usually kept in the medication room or on the medication cart. Others use a medication administration record (MAR), an 8½" × 11" chart. Still others use a combination of both. And an increasing number of facilities enter medication charting information into a computer, which automatically generates a list of administration times for all scheduled medication doses. Use of computers should help decrease the incidence of drug errors caused by misinterpretation of handwriting. (See *Computer-based pharmacy systems,* page 92, for more information.)

No matter what system a facility uses, Chapter 9 will show how to maintain medication records and accurately document medication administration. It will also explain how to report drug errors and how to use this information to promote quality assurance and prevent errors in the future.

Maintaining medication records

After the doctor writes a drug order, the nurse must verify the order by reviewing the drug, its therapeutic content, the dose (which may require checking the calculations), and the dosage form ordered. If a problem is detected, the nurse should contact the doctor before the drug order goes to the pharmacy. If the problem is not detected until after the drug order has gone to the pharmacy, the nurse must contact the doctor and the pharmacy.

Once the prescription has been verified, transcribe the order onto the medication charting form used in the facility. Drug order transcription requires close attention because a small error in rewriting an order can cause a major medication error.

Regardless of the type of medication charting form or system a facility uses, the nurse must record certain standard information. (See *Sample medication record,* page 93, for an example.) This information is required so that medication records can serve as legal documents, if necessary, to prove that a drug dose was given. All of this information must appear legibly in ink on the Kardex or MAR.

Computer-based pharmacy systems

As health care facilities purchase or develop computer systems, manufacturers offer increased choices among medication monitoring programs. In the simplest systems, the computer is used as a word processor or typewriter. The advantage of such a system is that the typed copy is easy to read, and the records can be stored on a disk in addition to, or instead of, hard (paper) copy.

More sophisticated systems provide listings of medications available in the facility's formulary. Doctors may have the option of selecting specific medications through various listings, such as pharmacologic categories, pharmacokinetic categories, and disease-related uses. Alternatively, medications may be ordered by typing a more traditional list, with those not in the facility's formulary being so identified at the time of the order. The doctor's order is sent to the facility's pharmacy for filling. The order also generates the patient's medication record, on which the nurse can document medication administration.

Such systems offer numerous advantages. As changes in medication orders are made, the pharmacy receives immediate notification, and the medication record is updated. This reduces the time required to request medications from the pharmacy and the time required to transcribe medications onto medication administration records. Errors from misinterpreted handwriting are eliminated. The availability of a medication is confirmed or denied immediately by the pharmacy.

Patient information

Record all patient information on the Kardex or MAR exactly as it appears on the patient's identification bracelet, stamping the Kardex or MAR with an admission data plate, if possible. If this is not available, write the patient's full name, hospital identification number, unit number, and bed assignment on the Kardex or MAR. Also include all known allergies, even those that are not drug related. If the patient has no known allergies, document this with the abbreviation NKA.

Dates

Certain dates must always appear on the Kardex or MAR: the date the prescription was written, the date the medication should begin (if different from the original order date), and the date the medication should be discontinued. In some facilities, the time the order is to be initiated is recorded with the date. This serves as a reference for the time to discontinue a drug when a limited period is indicated.

Drug information

As part of the medication charting information, include the drug name, strength, dosage form, and route of administration.

Drug name

Record the drug's full, preferably generic, name. If the doctor ordered the drug using a proprietary name, record this name as well. Avoid using abbreviations, chemical symbols, research names, and special institutional names, which could cause medication errors or delays in therapy.

Sample medication record

The medication Kardex below illustrates the kind of information required on all types of medication administration forms. Although different facilities may use different forms, the information is basically the same: patient information, date, drug information, time of administration, and the nurse's initials after administering the drug.

INITIAL	SIGNATURE	INITIAL	SIGNATURE
SA	Sally Adams RN		
JJ	Joan Johnson RN		

JOE JACKSON
33 SHORT STREET
HOPE N.J 2·21·24
UNIT : 4 SOUTH 432 A

ALLERGIES
  NKA

R = REFUSED O = OMITTED F = FASTING

DATE ORD.	STOP DATE	MEDICATION DOSE ROUTE FREQUENCY	R.N. INT.	HR.	2/14	2/15	2/16	2/17	2/18	2/19
2/14	2/19	carbidopa/levodopa (SINEMET) 25/250 P.O. Q.I.D	SA	A 10	X					
				P 2						
				P 6						
				P 10						
2/14	2/19	benztropine mesylate (COGENTIN) 1.0 mg P.O. T.I.D.	SA	A 10	X					
				P 2						
				P 6						
2/14	2/16	diphenhydramine hydrochloride (BENADYL) 25 mg. P.O. H.S.	SA	P 10						

FREEDOM HOSPITAL

ROUTINE MEDICATIONS

DIAGNOSIS & SURGERY: EXACERBATION PARKINSON

AGE: 64 SEX: M

PHYSICIAN: P.D. JONES

ROOM: 432A

NAME: JOE JACKSON

Drug strength

Be sure to document the actual amount of the drug to be administered.

Drug dosage form

Indicate the dosage form as ordered by the doctor. When recording the drug dosage form, consider the patient's special needs and the drug's physical form. For example, if a doctor orders sustained-action theophylline for a patient who has a nasogastric tube for chronic obstructive pulmonary disease, the patient could not take the tablets orally. The tablets would have to be crushed to be administered through the tube. But crushing sustained-action tablets would destroy the drug's integrity and alter its therapeutic action. In such a case, the nurse would have to contact the doctor to discuss and resolve the problem.

Route of administration

Always specify the route of administration. This is especially important for drugs that may be given by two different routes; for example, orally or rectally, as with acetaminophen (Tylenol). Some parenteral medications can be given by only one correct route; for example, NPH insulin may be given subcutaneously but not intravenously.

Time of administration

The doctor's order should include a desired administration schedule, such as t.i.d. or q6h. Transcribe it on the MAR and then convert it into actual times based on the facility's scheduled times (t.i.d. may be 9-1-5 in one facility and 10-2-6 in another), the availability and characteristics of the drug, or the drug's onset and duration of action (b.i.d. may be 10 and 6 or 10 and 10; q6h may be 4-10-4-10 or 6-12-6-12). Remember that time notations are based on a 24-hour clock, unless otherwise specified, and that the hour appearing *first* on a 24-hour clock should appear first in the time notation. So if an administration schedule is 2-10-2-10, the first 2 represents 2 A.M. (0200), the first 10 is 10 A.M. (1000), the second 2 is 2 P.M. (1400), and the second 10 is 10 P.M. (2200).

Some facilities have separate MARs or specially designated areas of the MAR for recording single drug orders or special drug orders (for example, drugs given as needed). Other facilities include these drugs on the daily MAR; in the latter case, the nurse must carefully distinguish these drugs from scheduled medications.

Initials

Usually, the person who transcribes the order to the MAR from the order sheet indicates this by signing the order sheet and initialing the order on the MAR. If someone other than a nurse transcribes the order, a nurse must co-sign the order sheet and the MAR.

Before administering medications, read the doctor's orders to ensure that the MAR accurately reflects the orders, including any recent orders or changes in orders. Many facilities require the nurse to initial the doctor's order sheet, on the line after the last order, to indicate that all orders have been transcribed correctly onto the MAR.

Maintaining medication records

Answer the following questions based on the *Sample medication record* on page 93. To check your answers, see page 99.

1. Which medications should be administered at 10:00 P.M.?

2. When should benztropine mesylate (Cogentin) be administered *next?*

3. What is the dosage and administration route for diphenhydramine hydro-chloride (Benadryl)?
4. Which medications should be administered at 6:00 P.M.?

Documenting medication administration

After administering a drug, the nurse may add to the MAR such information as missed doses or site of parenteral administration. If a dose is missed, the reason should also be documented in the progress notes. The nurse also should record the actual time of administration and should initial the record.

Dosage

If the dose administered varies in any way from the dose strength or amount ordered, note this fact in a special area on the MAR or in the patient's progress notes. For example, document whether the patient refused to take a medication, consumed only part of the medication, or vomited shortly after ingesting the medication.

Route of administration

When administering a drug by a parenteral route, record the injection site to facilitate site rotation. Most MAR forms include a numbered list of recognized sites so that the nurse can record the site by its number in the limited space available. If you administer a drug by a different route than that originally specified, indicate that change, along with the reason and authorization for the change.

Time of administration

Immediately after administering a drug, accurately document the time of administration to help prevent repeat administration of the same drug dose. For scheduled drugs (those with a planned time schedule), you will usually initial the appropriate time slot for the date you are giving the drug. Scheduled drug administration is considered on time if given within ½ hour before or after the ordered time. For unscheduled drugs (single doses, STATs, and p.r.n.s), indicate the exact time of administration in the appropriate slot. If a drug is not given as scheduled, be sure to document the reason for the delay or omission. Some MARs have a place for this information; others do not, requiring the information to be recorded in the patient's progress notes. Facility policy may require the nurse to initial and circle the particular time missed on the MAR to draw attention to the omission.

Identifying initials

The nurse who administers a drug must verify that the dose was given by initialing the MAR in the appropriate time slot. Make sure your initials are clearly legible and different from those of other nurses on the unit who might give drugs to the patient. (Use your middle initial for clarification, if necessary.) Then, identify your initials by recording them in the signature section of the MAR, along with your signature and title. Signature and initial identification must appear on every record that you initial when administering drugs. Always sign your initials in the same way on every record.

Other medication records

Some facilities require the nurse to document all drugs that a patient receives on a single Kardex or MAR. Other facilities use separate forms for p.r.n. drugs, large-volume parenterals, one-time-only doses, and treatment items (dermatologic and ophthalmic medications dispensed in bottles or tubes). Other medication records include perpetual inventory records and computerized records.

Perpetual inventory records

Federal and state laws regulate the dispensing, administering, and documenting of controlled substances. When a controlled substance is issued to a patient care area, it is accompanied by a perpetual inventory record on which the nurse documents the disposition of each dose.

If a doctor orders a controlled substance for a patient, record its administration on the Kardex or MAR and on the perpetual inventory record. When the dose is removed from the double-locked storage site, record the following information on the perpetual inventory record: the date and time the dose is removed, the patient's full name, the doctor's name, the drug's dose, and your signature. If any of the dose must be discarded, two nurses must verify the amount discarded and sign the form.

Computerized records

In a computerized records system, the computer generates a list of medications and administration times for each patient. After administering medication, use your password or sign-on code to enter the computer system, select the medications that were given, and note any medications that were not given, along with a reason why. When documenting parenteral medication administration, be sure to include their administration site.

With a computerized system, the nurse can enter the system at any time to determine which medications have already been — or need to be — administered. After 24 hours, a medical records clerk places a printout on the patient's chart. For each medication, the printout lists the dosage, administration route, time of administration, and person's name who administered it.

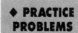

Documenting medication administration

Answer the following questions about documenting medication administration. (For questions 1 and 2, refer to the *Sample medication record* on page 93.) To check your answers, see page 99.

1. After administering medications to the patient at 2 P.M., the nurse should initial the 2-P.M. block for which medications?

2. After administering medications to the patient at 10 A.M., the nurse should place her initials in the 10-A.M. block for which medications?

3. At 2 P.M., a patient is vomiting and can't take the prescribed oral medications. Based on the key on the medication record, the nurse places an O next to the time when the medications were omitted. Is this documentation adequate?

4. After administering diphenhydramine hydrochloride (Benadryl) 50 mg I.M. at 10 P.M., as prescribed, the nurse initials the medication record in the appropriate block for 10 P.M. Is the documentation complete for this medication administration?

Assuring quality and preventing errors

Each facility has its own method for tracking medication administration errors. By tracking errors, the facility's quality assurance team can recommend ways to prevent future medication errors. One way to help ensure error-free medication administration is to become familiar with —

and carefully follow—facility policy, safety practices, and quality assurance recommendations.

Another way to prevent errors is to transcribe orders carefully from an order sheet to the MAR or Kardex. To avoid transcription errors, follow these guidelines:

- Transcribe all orders in a quiet, distraction-free area, if possible.
- Before signing the order sheet and initialing the MAR, carefully check all parts of the order.
- Follow facility policy for reviewing orders. Some facilities require that the nurse review all charts for new orders each shift and check any orders written within 24 hours. Other facilities give one shift (usually the night shift) the latter responsibility.

After medication administration, help prevent errors by making sure that the documentation is complete. Remember that the medication record should include the patient information, date, drug information, time of administration, and the nurse's initials. When medication is not given, be sure to document it on the medication record. If the MAR provides no space for this information, document it on the patient's progress notes.

◆ PRACTICE PROBLEMS

Assuring quality and preventing errors

Answer the following questions about assuring quality and preventing errors. To check your answers, see page 99.

1. By tracking medication errors, the _____ team can suggest ways to prevent future medication errors.

2. The nurse should carefully check all parts of the order before signing the _____ and initialing the MAR.

3. The nurse can avoid medication administration errors by making sure that _____ is complete.

4. The medication record should include the patient information, date, drug information, time of administration, and the nurse's _____ .

Reporting drug errors

Even when precautions are taken, errors in drug administration can occur. When they do, you need to report them by following these steps. If you make a drug administration error, report it to the doctor immediately. Also notify the pharmacist, who can provide information about drug interactions, dose-related problems (such as with an overdose or omitted dose), and antidotes, if needed. Then assess the patient, paying close attention to the drug's action and possible effects. Also remember to follow your facility's policies about documenting the event. For example, you may need to complete an incident report for legal purposes. Finally, supply all information required for follow-up by the quality assurance team.

◆ PRACTICE PROBLEMS

Reporting drug errors

Answer the following questions about reporting drug errors. To check your answers, see page 99.

1. When a drug error occurs, the nurse should immediately notify the _____ and the pharmacy.

2. If a drug error occurs, the nurse must continue to _____ the patient for any adverse effects.

3. For legal purposes, the nurse may need to complete an _____ report about a drug error.

Review problems

Answer the following questions about medication records. (For questions 1 through 9, refer to the medication record below.) To check your answers, see page 100.

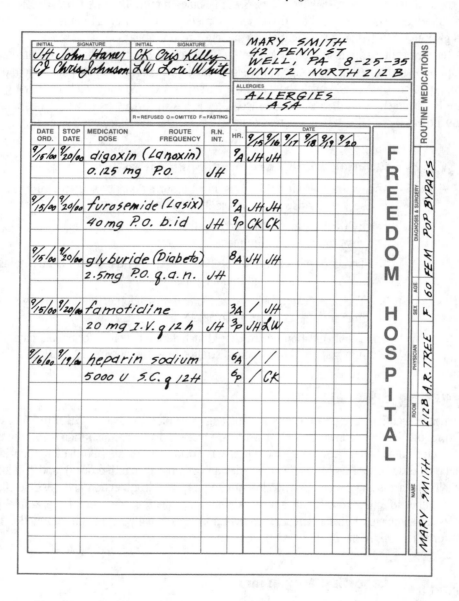

1. Which medications should be administered at 9 A.M.?
2. Which medication should be administered at 6 A.M.?
3. According to the medication record, can the nurse administer glyburide (DiaBeta) on 9/21?

4. By which route should the nurse administer digoxin (Lanoxin)?

5. Is this patient allergic to any medications?

6. Which medication should be administered at 6 P.M.?

7. The patient was supposed to receive furosemide (Lasix) 40 mg P.O. at 9 P.M. on 9/16. However, this dose was omitted as documented on the MAR. Is this documentation adequate?

8. After administering famotidine (Pepcid) as prescribed, the nurses initialed the appropriate blocks. Is their documentation complete?

9. Because surgery is scheduled at 10:00 A.M. on 9/17, the patient must remain NPO and miss the 8 A.M. and 9 A.M. doses of the prescribed oral medications on that day. How should the nurse document this on the MAR?

10. If a drug cannot be given as prescribed, the nurse should document the reason for this on the MAR or in the _____ .

11. When a drug error occurs, the nurse should notify the patient's doctor as well as the _____ .

12. When assessing the patient after a drug administration error, the nurse should pay close attention to the drug's _____ and possible effects.

13. Legally, an _____ should be filed for every drug error that occurs.

Answers to practice problems

◆ Maintaining medication records

1. carbidopa/levodopa (Sinemet) and diphenhydramine hydrochloride (Benadryl)

2. 6:00 P.M.

3. 25 mg P.O.

4. carbidopa/levodopa (Sinemet) and benztropine mesylate (Cogentin)

◆ Documenting medication administration

1. carbidopa/levodopa (Sinemet) and benztropine mesylate (Cogentin)

2. carbidopa/levodopa (Sinemet) and benztropine mesylate (Cogentin)

3. No. In addition to the O on the MAR, the nurse should document that the drug was omitted because the patient was vomiting. If the MAR has no space for this information, the nurse should document it in the progress notes.

4. No. For a parenteral medication, the nurse must also document the administration site.

◆ Assuring quality and preventing errors

1. quality assurance

2. order sheet

3. documentation

4. initials

◆ Reporting drug errors

1. doctor

2. assess

3. incident

Answers to review problems

1. digoxin (Lanoxin) and furosemide (Lasix)

2. heparin sodium

3. No. The stop date for glyburide (DiaBeta) is 9/20, so the nurse should not administer this drug on 9/21. The doctor must re-evaluate the order.

4. oral (P.O.) route

5. Yes. The patient is allergic to aspirin (ASA).

6. heparin sodium

7. No. The nurse should also state the reason for the omission in the patient's progress notes because the MAR provides no space for this information.

8. No. They should also document the administration site because famotidine is an I.V. drug.

9. When a patient does not receive medication because fasting is required, the nurse should write an F in the appropriate blocks and initial them. The nurse should also note this omission and its reason in the patient's progress notes.

10. progress notes

11. pharmacy

12. action

13. incident report

UNIT 4

Calculating Oral, Topical, and Rectal Dosages

Many facilities use the unit-dose system of drug distribution. This system provides drugs prepackaged in single-dose containers. Although the unit-dose system decreases the need for drug calculations, the nurse may encounter patient situations in which dosage calculations are necessary. In some instances, the calculations require conversions between systems of drug measurement. In others, they determine how many tablets, capsules, or other dosage forms to administer.

Unit 4 can prepare you for these responsibilities because the basic principles explained in its chapters apply to all oral, topical, or rectal medications. Chapter 10 explains how to read drug labels to obtain accurate information for all calculations. It provides examples of labels for oral drugs in tablet, capsule, and liquid form. Chapter 11 describes how to measure oral drugs and walks through the calculations needed to determine dosages of oral tablets, solutions, and powders. Chapter 12 demonstrates how to read labels for topical and rectal drugs. It also discusses dosage calculation and administration of these drugs.

As a nurse, you need to master all of these skills, to ensure patient safety when administering drugs by the oral, topical, or rectal route.

Chapter

10

♦

Oral Drug Labels

Before you can administer an oral drug safely, you must ensure that it is the proper drug and the proper dose. To do this, you must read its label carefully. Chapter 10 will show you how to read labels accurately for tablets, capsules, and oral solutions. It also will walk you through the steps involved in comparing the label to the patient's medication administration record (MAR) and safely administering the drug to the patient.

Reading tablet and capsule labels

Remember these three important words before administering every dose of medication: *Read the label.* Always know which drug you are to give, how much to administer, and why.

When reading any tablet or capsule label, particularly note the drug name, dosage strength, and expiration date.

Drug name

When reading the drug label the nurse should first check the generic name. If the drug has two names, the drug's generic name, usually appears in smaller print. The generic name is the accepted nonproprietary drug name, which is a simplified form of the drug's chemical name.

Next, note the drug's trade (brand or proprietary) name, if possible. This name, which is given by the manufacturer, is denoted by the registration ® symbol and usually appears first. Remember that a drug may have several different trade names, but only has one generic name. For example, the generic drug diazepam has many trade names, such as T-Quil, Valium, Valrelease, Vazepam, and Zetran. However, a drug may have only one name because it is so widely used and so well known by its generic name that the manufacturer did not need to develop a trade name. An example of this is atropine sulfate.

Be aware that the initials *U.S.P.* or *N.F.* may appear after the drug name. These abbreviations stand for two legally recognized standards for drugs: United States Pharmacopeia and National Formulary, respectively. A drug that is labeled U.S.P. or N.F. meets their standards for purity, potency, and storage, which are enforced by the Food and Drug Administration.

Some tablets or capsules actually contain two different drugs. The labels for these combination drugs list both generic names and their respective dosages. Such drugs are ordered by the trade name and the number of capsules or tablets to be administered, such as Percocet 1 tablet q4h p.r.n. pain. Review the following example to see how to read such as label.

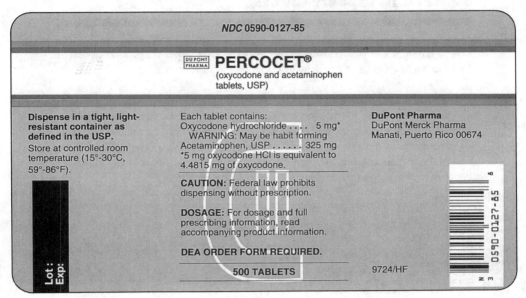

NDC 0590-0127-85

PERCOCET®
(oxycodone and acetaminophen tablets, USP)

Dispense in a tight, light-resistant container as defined in the USP.
Store at controlled room temperature (15°-30°C, 59°-86°F).

Each tablet contains:
Oxycodone hydrochloride . . . . 5 mg*
 WARNING: May be habit forming
Acetaminophen, USP . . . . . . 325 mg
*5 mg oxycodone HCl is equivalent to 4.4815 mg of oxycodone.

CAUTION: Federal law prohibits dispensing without prescription.

DOSAGE: For dosage and full prescribing information, read accompanying product information.

DEA ORDER FORM REQUIRED.

500 TABLETS

DuPont Pharma
DuPont Merck Pharma
Manati, Puerto Rico 00674

9724/HF

Lot :
Exp:

As this label states, Percocet contains oxycodone hydrochloride 5 mg and acetaminophen 325 mg. So instead of ordering it with a two-part dosage, the doctor prescribes it by the trade name Percocet and the number of tablets.

Dosage strength

After checking the drug name, look for the dosage strength on the label. Pay close attention to generic drugs because the labels and containers for different concentrations of the same drug may look exactly alike *except* for the listing of the drug's concentration. (See *Tablet and capsule labels,* pages 104 and 105, for examples of look-alike labels that the nurse must read carefully to avoid medication errors.)

Expiration date

Finally, be sure to check the expiration date. This vital piece of label information is often over-looked and needs to be given special attention. Expired drugs may be chemically unstable and may no longer provide the dose they were designed to deliver. If a drug has expired, return it to the pharmacy for proper disposal and for reimbursement of the patient.

Drug labels and drug orders

Safe drug administration requires comparing the doctor's order, as transcribed on the patient's MAR, *directly* against the drug label *three times* before administering the drug. The following example illustrates this procedure.

The MAR indicates that the patient is to receive propranolol hydrochloride (Inderal) 10 mg P.O. as part of the 10 A.M. medications. Open the patient's medication drawer, find the drug labeled propranolol hydrochloride (Inderal) 10 mg, and note that it is in oral tablet form. Then, place the labeled drug *directly* next to the transcribed order on the MAR, and carefully compare each part of the label and the order: propranolol hydrochloride, Inderal, and 10 mg.

Tablet and capsule labels

The following tablet and capsule labels illustrate look-alikes and sound-alikes that the nurse must read carefully to avoid medication errors.

Norpramin and norpace

On first glance, these medication names may be confused easily, which could lead to a medication error that could harm the patient. Norpramine is a tricyclic antidepressant, whereas Norpace is an antiarrhythmic. The inadvertent substitution of the antidepressant Norpramine for Norpace would not control the patient's arrhythmia, which could lead to serious complications.

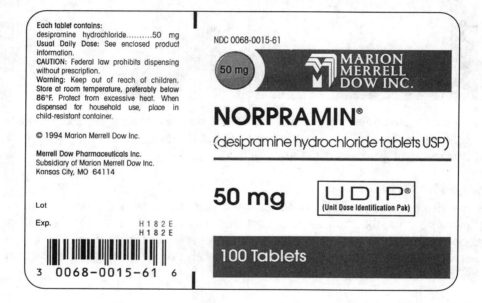

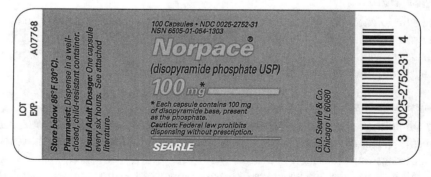

Tablet and capsule labels *(continued)*

Corgard

Although both of these bottles contain 100 Corgard tablets, they differ in one major way. The top bottle's tablets contain 20 mg each, and the bottom bottle's tablets contain 120 mg each—five times the dosage strength of the tablets on the top. If the bottles were accidentally interchanged, serious consequences could result.

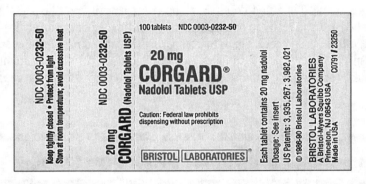

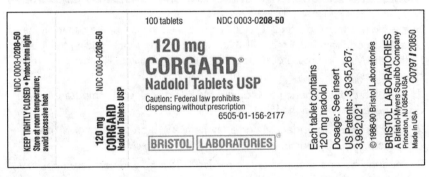

If the drug is supplied in bulk or in a stock bottle, transfer one tablet from the supply to a medication container, pouring from the supply to the lid and then into the container without handling the tablet. Before returning the supply to the drawer or shelf, once again compare the label to the order on the MAR and again note whether this is the right time for administration. Once a drug is removed from its container, you no longer can be certain that it is the correct drug—unless you have carefully compared the label to the MAR when pouring. At the bedside, positively identify the patient, administer the now-unlabeled drug, and record the administration. (See *Comparing a drug order with a drug label,* pages 106 and 107.)

Golden Rules

Before administering any drug, compare the drug order on the medication administration record against the drug label *three times.*

If the drug is supplied in a unit-dose packet, do *not* remove it from the packet until you are at the patient's bedside and ready to administer it. At that time, after positively identifying the patient, make the third drug check, again by comparing the label directly to the order before removing it from the packet. Be sure to note whether the time is correct for administering this drug. If so, administer the drug, and use the packet label for comparison when recording the administration.

Comparing a drug order with a drug label

Before administering a drug, carefully compare each part of the order on the medication administration record (MAR) with the drug label, holding the label next to the MAR to ensure accuracy. The following example illustrates the required steps.

1. Read the drug's generic name on the MAR (digoxin), and compare it to the drug's generic name on the label (digoxin).

2. Read the trade (proprietary) name on the MAR, if present (Lanoxin), and compare it to the proprietary name on the label (Lanoxin).

3. Read the dosage specified on the MAR (0.125 mg), and compare it to the dosage on the label (0.125 mg).

4. Read the route specified on the MAR (P.O.), and note the dosage form on the label (oral tablet).

5. Finally, note any special considerations on the MAR. (**Hold dose if apical pulse rate is < 56 beats/min and notify house officer.)

As a further safeguard, be sure to compare the MAR and drug label *three times* before actually administering the drug: once when obtaining the drug from floor stock or the patient's supply, a second time before placing the drug in the medication cup or other administration device, and a third time before either replacing the stock drug bottle on the shelf or removing the drug from the unit-dose packet at the patient's bedside.

Comparing a drug order with a drug label (continued)

Medication administration record

Any discrepancies between the MAR and the drug label require careful consideration. For instance, using the example below, suppose the MAR specified digoxin and the patient's drug packet was labeled only as Lanoxin; you would need to know that Lanoxin is a trade name for the drug digoxin. Suppose the drug packet was labeled digitoxin; you would need to recognize that this is a different digitalis glycoside that cannot be substituted for digoxin. Suppose the generic names were identical, but the packet contained a 0.25-mg tablet; you would have to know to administer one half of a tablet to achieve the required dosage. Remember, only through scrupulous attention to such details can the nurse ensure safe, error-free drug administration.

DATE ORD.	STOP DATE	MEDICATION DOSE — ROUTE FREQUENCY	R.N. INT.	HR.	DATE					
					8/8	8/9	8/10	8/11	8/12	8/13
8/8	8/11	digoxin (Lanoxin)	RY	A 10	X				X	D/C
		0.125 mg P.O. T.I.D. X		2P	LB				X	P̄
		11 doses		6P	JR AT-30				X	8/11
	**	HOLD DOSE IF APICAL								
		RATE < 56/min AND								
		NOTIFY HOUSE OFFICER								

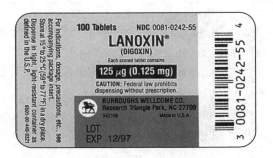

PRACTICE PROBLEMS

Reading tablet and capsule labels

Answer the following questions related to reading tablet and capsule labels. To check your answers, see page 114.

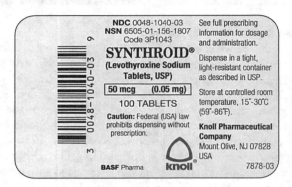

1. Answer these questions based on the label above.

a) What is the generic name?

b) What is the dosage strength?

c) What is the trade name?

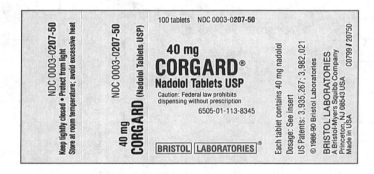

2. Answer these questions based on the label above.

a) What is the generic name?

b) What is the dosage strength?

c) What is the trade name?

3. Before administering a drug to a patient, the nurse should compare the drug label to the MAR _____ times.

4. If the drug comes in a _____ - _____ packet, the nurse should remove it at the bedside to ensure patient safety.

5. When comparing the drug to the patient's MAR, the nurse should note the drug's generic and trade names, _____ , _____ , dosage form, and special considerations.

Reading oral solution labels

In oral solutions, the dosage concentration is expressed as the weight of the drug (or dosage strength) contained in a volume of solution. For example, Lasix oral solution is provided as 10 mg/ml. Therefore, this oral solution contains 10 mg of Lasix (drug weight) in 1 ml (solution volume).

Keep in mind that oral solutions can also be measured in teaspoons, tablespoons, and ounces, but usually are measured in milliliters or cubic centimeters. Also remember to read oral solution labels carefully because the labels and containers for two different concentrations of the same drug sometimes look confusingly similar. (See *Oral solution labels* for examples.)

Oral solution labels

The following pairs of oral solution labels illustrate look-alikes that the nurse must read carefully to avoid medication errors.

Principen oral solution

These two containers both hold Principen oral solution. However, the top one contains 125 mg/5 ml, and the bottom one contains 250 mg/5 ml—twice the dosage concentration of the one on the top.

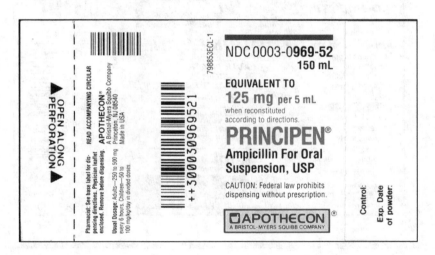

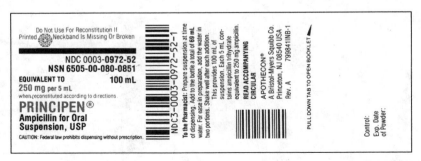

(continued)

Oral solution labels *(continued)*

Augmentin

These two containers are almost the same size, but the top container has a 5-ml dose of 125 mg, whereas the bottom one has a dose that's double this strength in the same volume of fluid—250 mg/5 ml.

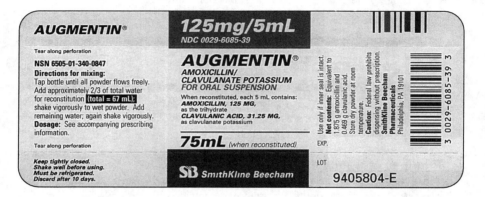

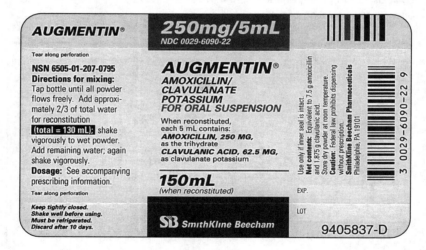

Oral solution labels (continued)

Mellaril

Although both of these bottles hold Mellaril, they differ in one major way. The drug concentration in the top bottle is 30 mg/1 ml; the concentration in the bottom bottle is 100 mg/1 ml. If these bottles were accidentally interchanged, serious consequences could result.

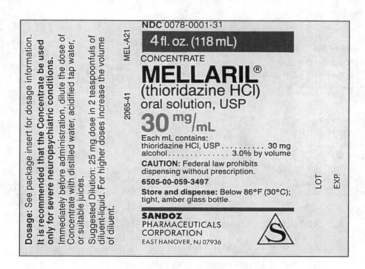

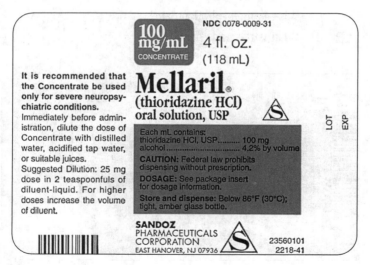

Reading oral solution labels

Answer the following questions related to reading oral solution labels. To check your answers, see page 115.

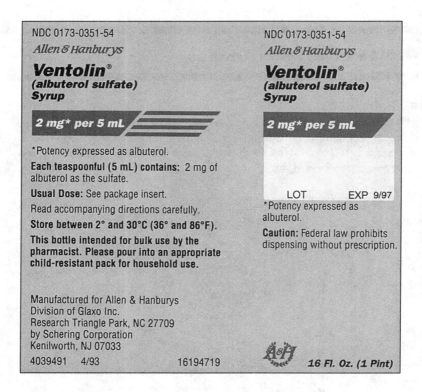

1. Answer these questions based on the label above.

   a) What is the generic name?

   b) What is the dosage concentration?

   c) What is the expiration date?

   d) What is the trade name?

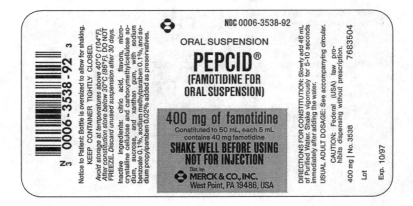

2. Answer these questions based on the label above.

   a) What is the generic name?

   b) What is the dosage concentration?

   c) What is the expiration date?

   d) What is the trade name?

Review problems

Answer the following questions related to oral drug labels. To check your answers, see page 115.

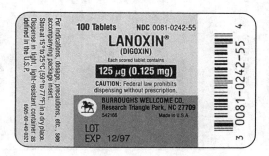

1. Answer these questions based on the label above.

   a) What is the generic name?

   b) What is the dosage strength?

   c) What is the expiration date?

   d) What is the trade name?

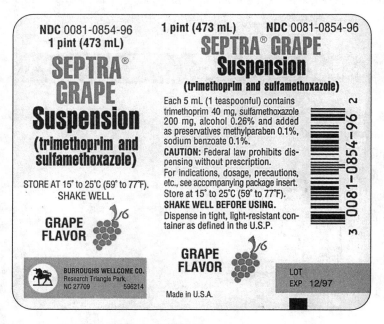

2. Answer these questions based on the label above.

   a) What is the generic name?

   b) What is the dosage concentration?

   c) What is the expiration date?

   d) What is the trade name?

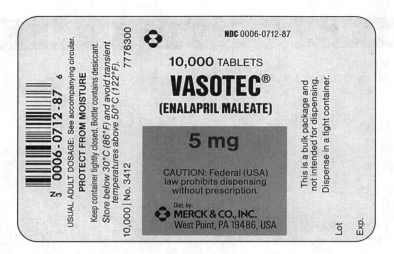

3. Answer these questions based on the label above.

   a) What is the generic name?

   b) What is the dosage strength?

   c) What is the trade name?

4. The nurse should check the drug's _____ name first when reading the label.

5. Why should the nurse check the label three times against the MAR before administering a drug?

Answers to practice problems

◆ Reading tablet and capsule labels

1. a) levothyroxine sodium

   b) 50 mcg

   c) Synthroid

2. a) nadolol

   b) 40 mg

   c) Corgard

3. three

4. unit-dose

5. dosage, route

◆ *Reading oral solution labels*

1. a) albuterol sulfate
   b) 2 mg per 5 ml
   c) 9/97
   d) Ventolin
2. a) famotidine
   b) 400 mg constituted to 50 ml; 40 mg per 5 ml after reconstitution
   c) 10/97
   d) Pepcid

Answers to review problems

1. a) digoxin
   b) 0.125 mg
   c) 12/97
   d) Lanoxin
2. a) trimethoprim and sulfamethoxazole
   b) trimethoprim 40 mg and sulfamethoxazole 200 mg/5 ml
   c) 10/97
   d) Septra Grape Suspension
3. a) enalapril maleate
   b) 5 mg
   c) Vasotec
4. generic
5. The nurse should compare the drug against the patient's MAR three times before administering it in order to ensure safe drug administration.

Chapter

11

◆ Oral Drug Dosage Calculation

To introduce you to dosage calculations, Chapter 11 begins with a review of ratios, fractions, and proportions. Then it shows how to calculate the correct dosage for tablets, capsules, oral solutions, and powders. It also demonstrates how to use measuring devices to obtain the correct dosage for administration. Throughout the chapter, practice problems offer opportunities to test and refine your calculation skills.

Many agencies use the unit-dose system of drug distribution. In this system, medications are packaged in single-dose containers, which facilitate drug distribution and administration. This ready-to-use form decreases the likelihood of errors because the medication remains in its labeled container until it is administered to the patient. (See *Unit-dose system* for more information.)

Although the unit-dose system of drug distribution decreases the need for drug calculations, the nurse may encounter patient situations in which dosage calculations are necessary. In some instances, the calculations require conversions between systems of drug measurement.

Unit-dose system

For many years, the nurse spent a great deal of time calculating doses and pouring medications, and these time-consuming tasks took away from other aspects of patient care. The use of the unit-dose drug distribution system has reduced this burden and has provided more time for evaluating patient responses to medications (desired and undesired) and for teaching patients about their drug regimens.

This timesaving system provides the exact dose of medication needed for each patient. In the unit-dose system, the pharmacist computes the number of tablets or the volume of liquid required and prepares the proper dose for administration. However, the nurse must still be able to perform the necessary calculations for measuring correct doses, because some facilities do not have unit-dose systems and others have systems that do not operate 24 hours a day.

In other instances, certain patients, such as those in critical care units or pediatric and geriatric patients, require individualized medication dosages. Some of these patients may need unusually small or large doses. Others need doses that are calculated to the nearest milligram instead of the nearest 10 mg. For these special patients, the *exact* individualized dose and the correct dosage calculation can mean the difference between a drug underdose and an overdose. (See Unit 6, Special Dosage Calculations, for details about pediatric and critical-care dosage calculations.)

Who are these special patients and what makes them need such highly individualized drug doses? Generally, they are patients whose ability to absorb, distribute, metabolize, or excrete drugs differs from that of normal individuals. Some of them cannot absorb drugs from the gastrointestinal (GI) tract because of upper GI disorders or surgery; deficiencies of gastric, pancreatic, or intestinal secretions; or passive congestion of GI blood vessels from severe congestive heart failure. These patients need drugs in parenteral form or in larger-than-average oral doses.

Patients with conditions that cause abnormal drug distribution from the GI tract or from parenteral sites to the sites of action also will need an altered dosing pattern. Premature infants and patients with low serum protein levels or severe liver or kidney disease cannot metabolize or excrete drugs as readily as normal patients and also will require alterations in drug doses.

The nurse can help individualize drug regimens for most of these patients by assessing kidney or liver function, monitoring blood levels of drugs, and calculating exact doses, as needed.

Calculating oral tablet dosages

Nurses and other health care professionals frequently use ratios or fractions in proportions to calculate drug dosages and to convert between measurement systems.

Review of ratios, fractions, and proportions

Because dosage calculations require that the nurse understands several mathematical concepts, this section reviews the basics of ratios, fractions, and proportions; describes how to apply them to many types of dosage calculations; and provides step-by-step examples of these procedures.

Terms and functions

Ratios and *fractions* are two ways to express the numerical relationship between two different things. A *proportion* is a mathematical statement that expresses equality between two ratios or two fractions. A proportion may be written using ratios, as in $1:3::2:6$, or using fractions, as in $\frac{1}{3} = \frac{2}{6}$.

When proportions are expressed using ratios, the product of the means equals the product of the extremes:

Proportion	Product of means and extremes
means	
$3:30::4:40$	$30 \times 4 = 3 \times 40$
extremes	

When proportions are expressed as fractions, their *cross products* are equal, as indicated below:

Proportion	Cross products
$\dfrac{2}{4} = \dfrac{5}{10}$	$2 \times 10 = 4 \times 5$

Whether ratios or fractions are used in a proportion, they must appear in the same order on both sides of the equal sign. When the proportion is expressed using ratios, the units of the first term on the left side of the equal sign must be the same as the units in the first term on the right side. In other words, the units of the mean on one side of the equal sign must match the units of the extreme on the other side, and vice versa. The example below demonstrates this principle.

mg : tablet :: mg : tablet

When the proportion is expressed using fractions, the units of measure in the numerators must be the same and the units of measure in the denominators must be the same. The example below demonstrates this principle.

$$\frac{mg}{tablet} = \frac{mg}{tablet}$$

Using proportions in dosage calculations. By keeping in mind a few rules, the nurse can avoid calculation errors that can lead to medication errors. In addition, these rules will simplify dosage calculations using proportions.

Leave units of measure in the calculation. This will help prevent one of the most common dosage calculation errors—the incorrect unit of measure. When the nurse leaves units of measure in the calculation, those in the numerator and the denominator cancel each other and leave the correct unit of measure in the answer, as in the following example.

Calculate how many milligrams of a drug are in two tablets if one tablet contains 4 mg.
◆ State the problem as a proportion.

4 mg : 1 tablet :: X mg : 2 tablets

◆ Solve for X by applying the principle that the product of the means equals the product of the extremes.

1 tablet × X mg = 4 mg × 2 tablets

◆ Divide and cancel the units of measure that appear in both the numerator and the denominator:

$$X = \frac{4 \text{ mg}}{1 \text{ tablet}} \times 2 \text{ tablets}$$

X = 8 mg

Watch the number of zeros and decimal places. An error in the number of zeros or decimal places in a calculation can cause a *tenfold* or greater dosage error.

The doctor orders 0.125 mg of digoxin P.O. The only digoxin on hand is a tablet that contains 0.25 mg. Calculate the number of tablets to administer.
◆ State the problem in a proportion.

0.25 mg : 1 tablet :: 0.125 mg : X tablet

◆ Solve for X.

1 tablet × 0.125 mg = 0.25 × X tablet

◆ Divide and cancel the units of measure that appear in both the numerator and denominator, carefully checking the decimal placement.

$$\frac{1 \text{ tablet}}{0.25 \text{ mg}} \times 0.125 \text{ mg} = X$$

X = 0.5 tablet

Recheck calculations that seem unusual. For example, if a calculation yields an answer that suggests administering 25 tablets or 200 ml of suspension, assume a calculation error and recheck the figures carefully. If you still have any doubt about your methods or results, review your calculations with another health care professional.

Use a calculator. Handheld calculators can improve the accuracy and speed of calculations. Remember, an electronic calculator cannot guarantee the accuracy of dosage calculations. The nurse must set up the proportions carefully and watch the units of measure and decimal places for the results to be reliable and accurate.

Determining the number of tablets or capsules to administer

Most tablets, capsules, and similar dosage forms are available in a few strengths only. The nurse usually will administer one tablet or one-half of a scored tablet. Breaking an unscored tablet in portions smaller than halves usually does not yield an accurate dose. If a dose smaller than one-half of a scored tablet or any portion of an unscored tablet is needed, the nurse should substitute a commercially available solution or suspension or one that is prepared by the pharmacist. Alternatively, the pharmacist could crush the tablet and weigh the exact dose. However, some oral preparations should not be opened, broken, scored, or crushed because that would change the drug's action. (See *Altering tablets and capsules* for detailed information.)

To calculate the number of tablets to administer, use the proportion method. The first ratio or fraction would be made up of the known tablet strength. The second ratio or fraction would contain the prescribed dose and the unknown quantity of tablets or capsules. Then solve for X to determine the proper number to administer.

Altering tablets and capsules

If a drug order requires you to break or crush a tablet or capsule, check first to see if this will affect the drug's action. Avoid crushing sustained-release (also called extended-, timed-, or controlled-release) drugs, although you may score and break some of them. Also avoid crushing capsules that contain tiny beads of medication, although you may empty the contents of some capsules into a beverage, pudding, or applesauce. Do not crush or score enteric-coated tablets, which usually appear shiny or glossy and are designed to protect the upper GI tract from irritation. Altering these tablets will cause GI upset. Also avoid altering buccal and sublingual tablets.

If you need to crush a tablet, use a chewable form, which is easier to crush. Then use a mortar and pestle or a pill crusher, or press the tablet between two spoons or place it in a small plastic bag and crush it with a rolling pin. Once the tablet is crushed, give the patient a drink to moisten the esophagus, and administer the crushed tablet with more water as soon as possible after crushing.

If you need to break a tablet, use one that is scored. Use a safe instrument, such as a spatula or a single-edged razor blade. If the tablet is unscored, it should be crushed and weighed and dispensed from the pharmacy in the correct weight dosage, because you cannot be certain that it will break into two even doses. You also should follow this procedure when you need to break a tablet into smaller pieces than the score allows or when you must administer a portion of a capsule. If the reason for crushing the tablet or opening the capsule is the patient's difficulty in swallowing the preparation, determine whether a liquid preparation of the same drug is available.

Patient situations

A drug order calls for propranolol 50 mg P.O. q.i.d., but the only available form of propranolol is 20-mg tablets. How many tablets must the nurse administer?

♦ Set up the first ratio with the known tablet strength.

$$20 \text{ mg} : 1 \text{ tab}$$

♦ Set up the second ratio with the desired dose and the unknown number of tablets.

$$50 \text{ mg} : X \text{ tab}$$

♦ Use these ratios in a proportion.

$$20 \text{ mg} : 1 \text{ tab} :: 50 \text{ mg} : X \text{ tab}$$

♦ Solve for X.

$$1 \text{ tab} \times 50 \text{ mg} = 20 \text{ mg} \times X \text{ tab}$$

$$X = \frac{1 \text{ tab} \times 50 \text{ mg}}{20 \text{ mg}}$$

$$X = 2\frac{1}{2} \text{ tablets}$$

A patient takes two 0.125-mg tablets of digoxin every morning. What is the equivalent dosage in milligrams?

♦ Set up a fraction with the known tablet strength.

$$\frac{0.125 \text{ mg}}{1 \text{ tab}}$$

♦ Set up a fraction with the unknown amount of milligrams and the dose the patient takes.

$$\frac{X \text{ mg}}{2 \text{ tab}}$$

♦ Use these fractions in a proportion, keeping similar terms in the same order on each side of the equal sign.

$$\frac{X \text{ mg}}{2 \text{ tab}} = \frac{0.125 \text{ mg}}{1 \text{ tab}}$$

♦ Solve for X.

$$X \text{ mg} \times 1 \text{ tab} = 2 \text{ tab} \times 0.125 \text{ mg}$$

$$X = \frac{2 \text{ tab} \times 0.125 \text{ mg}}{1 \text{ tab}}$$

$$X = 0.25 \text{ mg}$$

♦ **PRACTICE PROBLEMS**

Calculating oral tablet dosages

Answer the following questions about calculating oral tablet dosages. To check your answers, see page 129.

1. When a proportion is expressed using _____ , the units of measure in the numerators must be the same, and the units of measure in the denominators must be the same.

2. When a proportion is expressed using _____ , the units of the mean on one side of the equal sign must match the units of the extreme on the other side, and vice versa.

3. One tablet of furosemide contains 20 mg of the drug. Using a proportion with ratios, determine how many milligrams of furosemide are in three tablets.

4. The doctor prescribes ibuprofen 800 mg P.O. q6h, but only 400-mg tablets are available. How many tablets should the nurse administer?

5. A patient must receive Coumadin 10 mg P.O. at 6 P.M. The nurse has Coumadin 2.5-mg tablets on hand. How many tablets should the nurse administer?

6. The doctor prescribes Synthroid 175 mcg P.O. daily. However, the available tablets contain 25 mcg each. How many of these tablets should the nurse administer?

7. A patient must receive Corgard 240 mg P.O. daily, but only 40-mg tablets are available. How many tablets should the nurse administer?

8. For a diabetic patient, the doctor prescribes DiaBeta 1.25 mg P.O. daily. The nurse has 2.5-mg tablets available. How many tablets should the patient receive?

Calculating oral solution dosages

The nurse may need to administer medications in liquid form, either suspensions or elixirs. When handling any of these oral solutions, read the label carefully, being sure to identify the dosage strength contained in a particular amount of solution. Next, check the label for the expiration date. Then complete the dosage calculation, using the method of your choice.

Calculating the amount of solution to administer can be done using the proportion method. To do so, set up the first ratio or fraction with the known solution strength. Then set up the second ratio or fraction with the unknown quantity.

Patient situations

A patient is to receive 500 mg of amoxicillin oral suspension. The label reads AMOXI-CILLIN (Amoxicillin Trihydrate) 250 mg/5 ml, *and the bottle contains 100 ml. How many milliliters of amoxicillin solution should the patient receive?*

◆ Set up a fraction with the known solution strength.

$$\frac{5 \text{ ml}}{250 \text{ mg}}$$

◆ Set up a fraction with the unknown quantity.

$$\frac{X \text{ ml}}{500 \text{ mg}}$$

◆ Set up the proportion and solve for X.

$$\frac{X \text{ ml}}{500 \text{ mg}} = \frac{5 \text{ ml}}{250 \text{ mg}}$$

$$X \text{ ml} \times 250 \text{ mg} = 500 \text{ mg} \times 5 \text{ ml}$$

$$X = \frac{500 \text{ mg} \times 5 \text{ ml}}{250 \text{ mg}}$$

$$X = 10 \text{ ml}$$

Oxacillin suspension for oral administration contains 500 mg/5 ml. Based on this information from the drug label, calculate the volume needed to administer a 300-mg dose, using ratios and the proportion method.

♦ Set up the ratios of the known and unknown solution strengths.

$$500 \text{ mg} : 5 \text{ ml} :: 300 \text{ mg} : X \text{ ml}$$

♦ Solve for X.

$$5 \text{ ml} \times 300 \text{ mg} = 500 \text{ mg} \times X \text{ ml}$$

$$X = \frac{5 \text{ ml} \times 300 \text{ mg}}{500 \text{ mg}}$$

$$X = 3 \text{ ml}$$

Calculating dosages with oral powders

Drugs that are unstable when stored as liquids are supplied in powder form. Before administering such a drug to a patient, dilute it with the appropriate diluent, or liquid used for dilution. (The usual diluent for oral drugs is tap water.) Be sure to read the drug label to determine how much diluent to add. After adding the diluent, read the label again to determine the dosage strength contained in the volume of fluid. Then apply the same dosage calculations that you would use to calculate other oral solution dosages.

Measuring oral solutions

To administer an oral solution accurately, you should measure it with a medication cup, dropper, or syringe. Medicine cups are calibrated to measure solutions in milliliters, tablespoons, teaspoons, drams, and ounces. To accurately measure an oral solution, hold the cup at eye level while pouring the solution. Drugs that are prescribed in drops usually are packaged with a dropper. If not, you can use a standard dropper as a substitute. Oral syringes are easy to identify because—unlike other syringes—their tips are off center. They can be used to measure oral solutions in milliliters or teaspoons.

After measuring and administering a drug from a multiple-dose container, remember to store it as directed on the drug label.

Calculating oral solution dosages

Calculate the following oral solution dosages. To check your answers, see page 129.

1. The doctor prescribes Zovirax suspension 400 mg P.O. b.i.d. The label states that each 5 ml contains 200 mg. How many milliliters should the nurse administer?

2. A patient must receive Pepcid oral suspension 20 mg P.O. daily h.s. The solution contains 40 mg/5 ml. How many milliliters of solution should the patient receive?

3. A drug order reads *Dilantin oral suspension 100 mg P.O. b.i.d.* The oral suspension contains 125 mg/5 ml. How many milliliters should the nurse administer with each dose?

4. The doctor prescribes Ceclor oral suspension 500 mg P.O. q8h. The drug label reads 125 mg/5 ml. How many milliliters should the nurse administer with each dose?

5. A patient needs to receive Lasix oral solution 80 mg P.O. daily. The label states that the solution contains 10 mg/ml. How many milliliters should the patient receive?

6. The nurse has just reconstituted Suprax oral powder with 69 ml of water, as directed on the label, to obtain 100 ml of Suprax suspension. The dosage strength of the reconstituted solution is 100 mg/5 ml. For a patient with a urinary tract infection, the doctor has ordered Suprax 400 mg P.O. daily. How many milliliters of the suspension should the patient receive?

7. When using a medication cup to measure a drug dose, the nurse should hold the cup at _____ _____ .

8. After administering a drug from a multiple-dose container, the nurse should store it as directed on the _____ _____ .

Performing two-step dosage calculations

Most dosage calculations require more than one equation. For example, medications may be ordered in one system of measurement but may be available in tablet, capsule, or liquid form in another system of measurement. In these situations, the nurse must convert from one system to another and then determine the number of capsules or tablets or the amount of solution to administer.

This section describes how to perform complete dosage calculations based on drug order and drug label information, using ratios and fractions in proportions. In addition, it offers two alternative approaches: the "desired-over-have" and the "ordered-available" methods of solving two-step dosage calculations.

Basic guidelines

Use the following guidelines to determine the number of capsules or tablets or the amount of solution to be given to the patient when the medication is ordered in a measurement system different from the one available.

◆ Read the drug order thoroughly, paying close attention to decimal places and zeros.

◆ Convert the dose from the system in which it is ordered to the system in which it is available.

◆ Calculate the number of capsules or tablets or the amount of solution needed to obtain the desired dose.

Patient situations

The doctor's order states **Lithium carbonate gr XX P.O. t.i.d.** *The drug label states* **Lithium Carbonate USP 300 mg/capsule.** *How many capsules should the nurse give to the patient for one dose?*

◆ Convert gr XX, 20 grains, from the system in which it is ordered to the metric system, using fractions in a proportion and standard equivalents. (See *Equivalent measures*, page 73.)

$$\frac{X \text{ mg}}{20 \text{ gr}} = \frac{60 \text{ mg}}{1 \text{ gr}}$$

◆ Solve for X.

$$X \text{ mg} \times 1 \text{ gr} = 20 \text{ gr} \times 60 \text{ mg}$$

$$X = \frac{20 \text{ gr} \times 60 \text{ mg}}{1 \text{ gr}}$$

$$X = 1,200 \text{ mg}$$

♦ The dose to be administered is 1,200 mg. Determine the number of capsules to administer by setting up a proportion.

$$\frac{X \text{ cap}}{1,200 \text{ mg}} = \frac{1 \text{ cap}}{300 \text{ mg}}$$

♦ Solve for X.

$$X \text{ cap} \times 300 \text{ mg} = 1,200 \text{ mg} \times 1 \text{ cap}$$

$$X = \frac{1,200 \text{ mg} \times 1 \text{ cap}}{300 \text{ mg}}$$

$$X = 4 \text{ capsules}$$

A drug order calls for digoxin pediatric elixir 0.25 mg P.O. once daily. According to the label on the bottle, the solution contains 50 mcg/ml. How much elixir should the nurse administer?

♦ Convert milligrams to micrograms (1 mg = 1,000 mcg).

$$1 \text{ mg} : 1,000 \text{ mcg} :: 0.25 \text{ mg} : X \text{ mcg}$$

$$1,000 \text{ mcg} \times 0.25 \text{ mg} = 1 \text{ mg} \times X \text{ mcg}$$

$$X = \frac{1,000 \text{ mcg} \times 0.25 \text{ mg}}{1 \text{ mg}}$$

$$X = 250 \text{ mcg}$$

♦ Calculate the volume of elixir to administer.

$$50 \text{ mcg} : 1 \text{ ml} :: 250 \text{ mcg} : X \text{ ml}$$

$$1 \text{ ml} \times 250 \text{ mcg} = 50 \text{ mcg} \times X \text{ ml}$$

$$X = \frac{1 \text{ ml} \times 250 \text{ mcg}}{50 \text{ mcg}}$$

$$X = 5 \text{ ml}$$

This drug comes with a special dropper calibrated in micrograms and milliliters. Read the calibration marks carefully when administering this drug because it has a narrow therapeutic margin.

Desired-over-have method

Desired-over-have and ordered-available methods offer alternative ways to solve two-step problems. Desired-over-have uses the proportion method already described and also follows two steps; ordered-available incorporates two steps into one equation.

Desired-over-have uses fractions to express known and unknown quantities.

$$\frac{\text{Desired units}}{\text{Have units (X)}} = \text{Equivalent} \frac{\text{(Same units as Desired)}}{\text{(Same units as Have)}}$$

Patient situation

Twenty mEq of potassium chloride are ordered and a solution containing 10 mEq potassium chloride/5 ml is available. How many milliliters should the nurse administer?

♦ Set up the equation to express known and unknown quantities.

$$\frac{X \text{ ml desired}}{5 \text{ ml have}} = \frac{20 \text{ mEq desired}}{10 \text{ mEq have}}$$

♦ Solve for X.

$$X \text{ ml} \times 10 \text{ mEq} = 5 \text{ ml} \times 20 \text{ mEq}$$

$$X = \frac{5 \text{ ml} \times 20 \text{ mEq}}{10 \text{ mEq}}$$

$$X = 10 \text{ ml}$$

Ordered-available method

The ordered-available method uses only one equation to convert between systems of measurement and to calculate the amount of medication to administer. However, this method requires caution. If any part of the equation is misplaced (such as placing a quantity in the numerator that should be in the denominator), the error may not be immediately apparent and could lead to significant errors in calculation.

$$X \text{ tab} = \text{ordered dose} \times \text{conversion factor} \times \frac{\text{available amount of dosage form}}{\text{quantity of drug per dosage form}}$$

Multiply the ordered dose by the conversion factor, then by a fraction expressing the quantity of drug per unit of dosage form (tablets, capsules, etc.). When setting up the equation, the nurse must take care to have the denominator of the conversion factor be in the same units as the ordered dose. If the equation is set up correctly, all units will cancel each other, leaving only the amount sought.

Patient situation

A patient is to receive 0.25 mg of Synthroid P.O. The pharmacy supplies the drug in tablets that contain 125 mcg each. How many tablets should the nurse administer?

♦ Multiply the conversion factor 1,000 mcg = 1 mg. Remember to make the fraction's denominator the same unit as the ordered dose (mg). Then multiply by a fraction, expressing the amount of the drug in 1 tablet.

$$X \text{ tablets} = 0.25 \text{ mg} \times \frac{1,000 \text{ mcg}}{1 \text{ mg}} \times \frac{1 \text{ tablet}}{125 \text{ mcg}}$$

$$X = 2 \text{ tablets}$$

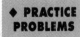 **♦ PRACTICE PROBLEMS**

Performing two-step dosage calculations

Perform the following dosage calculations, using the two-step method of your choice. To check your answers, see page 129.

1. If a drug order calls for Kaon-CL liquid 40 mEq and the preparation contains 20 mEq/15 ml, how many tablespoons would deliver the same dose?

2. If a patient takes 1 tsp of Tagamet and the drug contains 300 mg/5 ml, how many milligrams does the patient receive with each dose?

3. How many teaspoons of a 325 mg/5 ml elixir would a nurse give to deliver 650 mg of Tylenol?

4. The doctor orders 1 g of ampicillin P.O. q6h; 500 mg capsules are available. How many capsules should the patient receive with each dose?

5. A patient requires 62.5 mcg of digoxin elixir P.O. daily. The elixir contains 0.05 mg/ml. How many milliliters of the drug does the patient need?

Review problems

Perform the following dosage calculations for oral drugs. To check your answers, see page 130.

1. The doctor prescribes Prinivil 40 mg P.O. daily. The label on the bottle is:

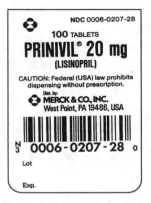

How many tablets should the nurse administer?

2. The doctor prescribes Zocor 10 mg P.O. daily at 6 P.M. The label on the bottle is:

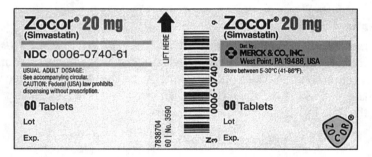

How many tablets should the nurse administer?

3. The doctor prescribes Coumadin 7.5 mg P.O. daily. The label on the bottle is:

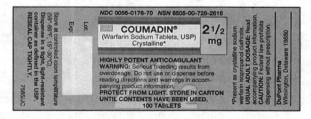

How many tablets should the nurse administer?

4. The doctor prescribes Norpramin 50 mg P.O. daily. The label on the bottle is:

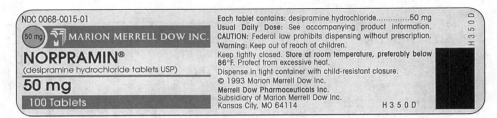

How many tablets should the nurse administer?

5. If a drug order calls for 30 mg of propranolol but the only available form is 20-mg tablets, how many tablets should the nurse administer?

6. Hydroxyzine hydrochloride is available in 10-mg tablets but the drug order calls for a 20-mg dose. How many tablets make up that dose?

7. Chlorothiazide is available in 500-mg tablets, but the drug order calls for a 750-mg dose. How many tablets should the nurse administer?

8. If Hexadrol is available in 1.5-mg tablets but the drug order calls for a 6-mg dose, how many tablets should the nurse administer?

9. Cylert is available in 37.5-mg tablets but the drug order calls for a 56.25-mg dose. How many tablets make up that dose?

10. If Synthroid is available in 100-mcg tablets but the drug order calls for a 250-mcg dose, how many tablets should the nurse administer?

11. The doctor prescribes Zantac syrup 150 mg P.O. b.i.d. The label on the bottle is:

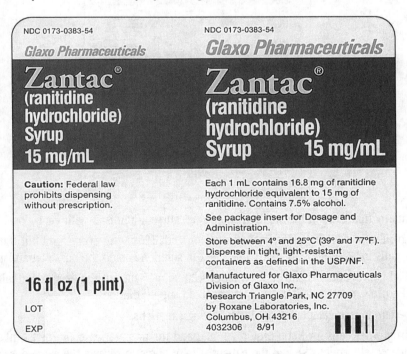

How many milliliters of the solution need to be given with each dose?

12. The doctor prescribes Augmentin oral suspension 250 mg P.O. q8h. The label on the bottle is:

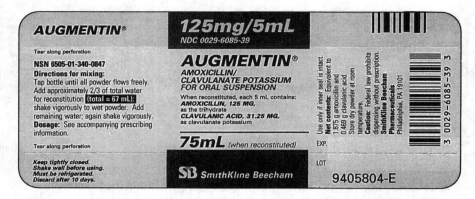

How many milliliters of the solution would provide that dose?

13. The doctor prescribes prednisone oral solution 15 mg P.O. b.i.d. The label on the bottle is:

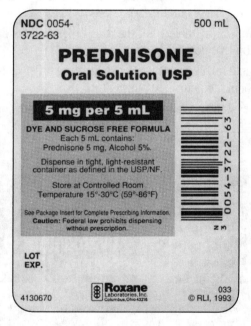

How many milliliters of the solution should the nurse administer with each dose?

14. If ampicillin is available as an oral suspension with 125 mg in every 5 ml but the drug order calls for 250 mg, how many milliliters of solution should the nurse administer?

15. Kay Ciel is available for oral replacement as 20 mEq/15 ml but the drug order calls for 10 mEq. How many milliliters of solution would supply that dose?

Use a two-step dosage calculation for the following situations.

16. If a drug order calls for Kaon Liquid 20 mEq and the preparation contains 20 mEq/15 ml, how many tablespoons should the patient take at home to receive the same dose?

17. If a patient has been taking 2 tsp of Tagamet with each meal, and the drug contains 300 mg/5 ml, how many milligrams has the patient received with each dose?

18. For a child, the doctor prescribes triprolidine hydrochloride 1.25 mg P.O. q6h. The oral preparation contains 1.25 mg/5 ml. How many teaspoons will the nurse instruct the child's parents to administer for each dose?

19. How many teaspoons of a 250 mg/5 ml suspension should a patient take to consume 500 mg of amoxicillin trihydrate?

20. How many milliequivalents of potassium are in 1 tsp of solution labeled *Potassium gluconate 20 mEq/15 ml*?

Answers to practice problems

◆ Calculating oral tablet dosages

1. fractions

2. ratios

3. 20 mg : 1 tablet :: X mg : 3 tablets
   X = 20 × 3
   X = 60 mg

4. 2 tablets

5. 4 tablets

6. 7 tablets

7. 6 tablets

8. ½ tablet

◆ Calculating oral solution dosages

1. 10 ml

2. 2.5 ml

3. 4 ml

4. 20 ml

5. 8 ml

6. 20 ml

7. eye level

8. drug label

◆ Performing two-step dosage calculations

1. 2 Tbs

2. 300 mg

3. 2 tsp

4. 2 capsules

5. 1.25 ml

Answers to review problems

1. 2 tablets
2. ½ tablet
3. 3 tablets
4. 1 tablet
5. 1½ tablets
6. 2 tablets
7. 1½ tablets
8. 4 tablets
9. 1½ tablets
10. 2½ tablets
11. 10 ml
12. 10 ml
13. 15 ml
14. 10 ml
15. 7.5 ml
16. 1 Tbs
17. 600 mg
18. 1 tsp
19. 2 tsp
20. 6.67 mEq

Chapter

12

◆

Topical and Rectal Medications

Some medications must be administered by the topical (or dermal) route. Topical medications include creams, lotions, ointments, powders, and patches. Each form has special considerations that the nurse must understand to ensure safe administration. So Chapter 12 presents the most common topical drugs and describes how to administer them safely.

Medications may be given by the rectal route for various reasons. This route may be preferred in a patient who can't take drugs orally, such as one with a nasogastric tube or with nausea or vomiting. It may also be the preferred route in a patient who is unconscious and can't swallow or who needs certain local and systemic effects (such as from bisacodyl suppositories that are given for constipation). This chapter introduces rectal medications, such as suppositories, and demonstrates how to perform related dosage calculations.

Reading topical and rectal drug labels

Reading the labels on topical medications and rectal suppositories is much like reading the labels on oral and parenteral medications. If the drug has a trade name, it appears first. It is followed by the generic name, dosage strength, and total volume of the package. Some labels also contain special instructions about administration. (See *Topical and rectal drug labels,* page 132, for examples.)

Topical and rectal drug labels

When reading a topical ointment label, note the following information as shown on this box label:
- ◆ Trade name, which is Bactroban
- ◆ Generic name, which is mupirocin ointment 2%
- ◆ Dosage strength, which is 2% ointment
- ◆ Total package volume, which is 15 grams
- ◆ Special instructions, which are not included on the front of this label.

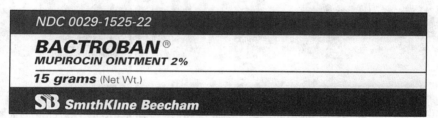

When reading a rectal suppository label, note the following information as shown on this box label:
- ◆ Trade name, which is Compazine
- ◆ Generic name, which is prochlorperazine suppositories
- ◆ Dosage strength, which is 5 mg per suppository
- ◆ Total package volume, which is 12 suppositories
- ◆ Special instructions, which are "For older children (not under 40 lb). For rectal use only."

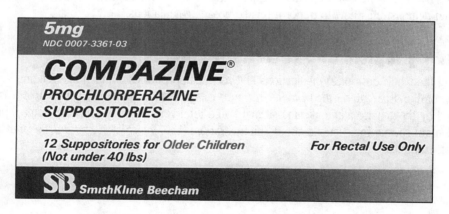

◆ PRACTICE PROBLEMS

Reading topical and rectal drug labels

Answer the following questions about topical and rectal drug labels. To check your answers, see page 138.

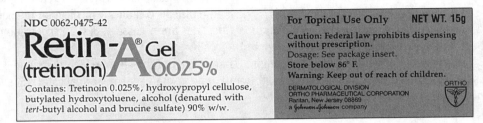

1. Based on the topical drug label above, answer these questions.
   a) What is the drug's trade name?
   b) What is the drug's generic name?
   c) What is the dosage strength?
   d) What is the total volume of the package?

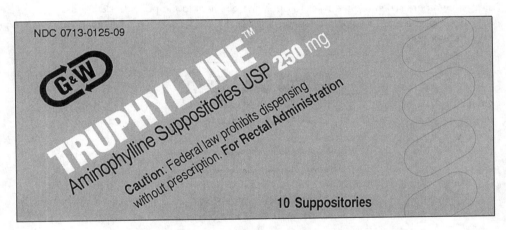

2. Based on the rectal drug label above, answer these questions.
   a) What is the drug's trade name?
   b) What is the drug's generic name?
   c) What is the dosage strength?
   d) What special instructions appear on the label?

Calculating dosages

The nurse calculates dosages for topical drugs and rectal suppositories using different techniques from those used for oral and parenteral medications.

Topical drugs

Topical drugs are administered by the dermal route. This means that they are applied to the skin and absorbed through the epidermal layer into the dermis. Most topical drugs are used for their local effects, rather than their systemic effects. A few, such as nitroglycerin, are used for their systemic effects.

Topical drugs include creams, lotions, ointments, powders, and patches. Because they are commonly prescribed, use of ointments and patches is described in detail.

When the doctor prescribes an ointment as part of wound care or dermatologic treatment, the amount to apply usually is left to the nurse's judgment, occasionally with such general guidance as "use a thin layer" or "apply thickly." When an ointment contains a medication intended for a systemic effect, more specific administration guidelines are necessary. Several medications that act on the cardiovascular system are applied topically.

Nitroglycerin ointment, used to treat angina, is available in tubes from which the nurse measures the correct dose. To apply ointment from a tube, use a paper ruler applicator. (See *Using a paper ruler applicator* for details.)

Using a paper ruler applicator

To measure a specified amount of ointment from a tube, squeeze the prescribed length of ointment (in inches or centimeters) onto a paper ruler like the one shown here. Then use the ruler to apply the ointment to the patient's skin at the appropriate time, following the pharmaceutical manufacturer's guidelines for administration.

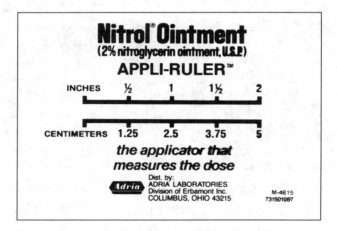

Nitroglycerin also comes in sustained-release transdermal patches. To apply a transdermal nitroglycerin patch, remove the previously applied patch and replace it with the new patch at the appropriate time, following the manufacturer's guidelines for administration.

Other drugs are available in patches that deliver the dose over a period of time. These include fentanyl, clonidine hydrochloride, and estrogen. The fentanyl transdermal system (Duragesic patch) is used to manage chronic pain. It holds the drug in a reservoir behind a membrane that allows controlled drug absorption through the skin. It is available in 25, 50, 75, and 100 mcg/hour; the higher dosages are used for opioid-resistant patients. To ensure that the patient receives the correct dosage, change the patch every 72 hours, check the label to verify the fentanyl dosage, and note the size and color of the patch. Patch size increases and patch color changes as the dosage increases.

Rectal drugs

Rectal drugs include enemas and suppositories. Because suppositories are the most common form, they are the focus of this section. Suppositories are useful for patients who cannot take medications orally. As with oral drugs, however, the nurse calculates the number of suppositories to administer by using the proportion method with ratios or fractions. Although the doctor usually prescribes drugs in the dosage provided by one suppository, two suppositories occasionally are needed. However, the nurse should always recheck calculations that indicate more than one suppository is needed. Also contact the pharmacy to determine whether the medicated suppository is available in other dosage strengths. If more than two suppositories are needed to provide one dose, contact the doctor.

Patient situations

A child is to receive 60 mg of pentobarbital via suppository. The package label reads **Nembutal sodium suppositories (pentobarbital sodium suppositories).** *Each suppository contains 30 mg of pentobarbital sodium. How many suppositories should the nurse administer?*

◆ Set up the proportion.

$$\frac{X \text{ supp}}{60 \text{ mg}} = \frac{1 \text{ supp}}{30 \text{ mg}}$$

◆ Solve for X.

$$X \text{ supp} \times 30 \text{ mg} = 60 \text{ mg} \times 1 \text{ supp}$$
$$X = \frac{60 \text{ mg} \times 1 \text{ supp}}{30 \text{ mg}}$$
$$X = 2 \text{ suppositories}$$

If, in the above example, each suppository contains 15 mg of pentobarbital sodium, how many suppositories should the nurse give to the patient?

◆ Set up the proportion.

$$\frac{X \text{ supp}}{60 \text{ mg}} = \frac{1 \text{ supp}}{15 \text{ mg}}$$

◆ Solve for X.

$$X \text{ supp} \times 15 \text{ mg} = 60 \text{ mg} \times 1 \text{ supp}$$
$$X = \frac{60 \text{ mg} \times 1 \text{ supp}}{15 \text{ mg}}$$
$$X = 4 \text{ suppositories}$$

Because more than one Nembutal suppository is needed, the nurse should recheck the calculations and also have another nurse perform the calculations. Next, after again determining that four suppositories should be given and noting that 60 mg is a safe dose of Nembutal for a child, the nurse should contact the pharmacy. The pharmacist would know that Nembutal is available in suppositories containing 30, 60, 120, and 200 mg. By using a 60-mg suppository, the nurse would be able to give the child one rather than four.

If, in the same example, the patient was to receive 15 mg of pentobarbital and each suppository contained 30 mg, how many suppositories would the nurse give to the patient?
◆ Set up the proportion.

$$\frac{X \text{ supp}}{15 \text{ mg}} = \frac{1 \text{ supp}}{30 \text{ mg}}$$

◆ Solve for X.

$$X \text{ supp} \times 30 \text{ mg} = 15 \text{ mg} \times 1 \text{ supp}$$

$$X = \frac{15 \text{ mg} \times 1 \text{ supp}}{30 \text{ mg}}$$

$$X = 0.5 \text{ suppository}$$

Because less than one Nembutal suppository is needed, the nurse should recheck the calculations and also have another nurse perform the calculations. Rather than give half of the available 30-mg suppository, contact the pharmacy to order Nembutal in a 15-mg suppository, if available.

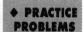

Calculating dosages

Perform the following calculations related to topical and rectal drugs. To check your answers, see page 138.

1. When a doctor prescribes ointments as a part of wound care or as a dermatologic treatment, the amount to apply usually is left to the _____ judgment.

2. The doctor's order reads: *Nitrol ointment 1″ q6h.* How should the nurse measure this dose?

3. A topical patch holds the drug in a reservoir behind a membrane that allows controlled drug _____ through the skin.

4. If a patient needs ASA 120 mg by suppository daily, and ASA 60 mg suppositories are available, how many suppositories should the nurse administer?

5. A drug order reads: *Tigan 400 mg per rectum.* On hand are 200-mg suppositories. How many should the nurse give?

6. If a patient needs to receive Compazine 25 mg rectally, and 25-mg suppositories of Compazine are available, how many suppositories should the nurse administer?

7. A drug order reads: *chlorpromazine hydrochloride 200 mg per rectum.* On hand are 100-mg suppositories. How many suppositories should the nurse administer?

8. If a patient needs bisacodyl 10 mg, and 5-mg suppositories are available, how many suppositories should the nurse administer?

Review problems

Answer the following questions about topical and rectal drugs and dosage calculations. To check your answers, see page 138.

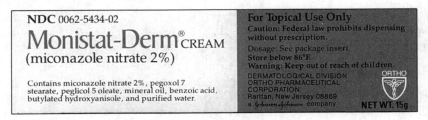

NDC 0062-5434-02

Monistat-Derm®CREAM
(miconazole nitrate 2%)

Contains miconazole nitrate 2%, pegoxol 7 stearate, peglicol 5 oleate, mineral oil, benzoic acid, butylated hydroxyanisole, and purified water.

For Topical Use Only
Caution: Federal law prohibits dispensing without prescription.
Dosage: See package insert.
Store below 86°F.
Warning: Keep out of reach of children.
DERMATOLOGICAL DIVISION
ORTHO PHARMACEUTICAL CORPORATION
Raritan, New Jersey 08869
a Johnson&Johnson company
ORTHO
NET WT. 15g

1. Based on the topical drug label above, answer these questions.

    a) What is the drug's trade name?

    b) What is the drug's generic name?

    c) What is the dosage strength?

2. For a patient with abrasions from a motor vehicle accident, the doctor prescribes bacitracin ointment to be applied to the abrasions. How much ointment should the nurse apply?

3. The doctor prescribes Nitrol (nitroglycerin) ointment 1½″ for a patient. How should the nurse measure this dose before administering it?

4. A patient needs to receive 250 mg of aminophylline. The label lists the contents as *Aminophylline suppositories USP 250 mg per suppository.* How many suppositories should the patient receive?

5. A patient must receive trimethobenzamide hydrochloride (Tigan) 200 mg by rectal suppository. The pharmacy has 100-mg suppositories available. How many suppositories should the nurse administer?

6. A patient is to receive indomethacin (Indocin) 25 mg P.R. b.i.d. The nurse has 50-mg suppositories available. How many suppositories should the nurse administer?

7. A child must receive morphine sulfate 2.5 mg P.R. The nurse has 5-mg suppositories on hand. How many suppositories should the child receive?

8. The doctor prescribes thiethylperazine maleate (Norzine) 10 mg P.R. The pharmacy supplies the drug in a 10-mg suppository. How many suppositories should the nurse administer?

Answers to practice problems

◆ Reading topical and rectal drug labels

1. a) Retin-A Gel
   b) tretinoin
   c) 0.025% ointment
   d) 15 grams
2. a) Truphylline
   b) aminophylline suppositories USP
   c) 250 mg/suppository
   d) Federal law prohibits dispensing without prescription. For rectal administration.

◆ Calculating dosages

1. nurse's
2. The nurse should measure 1″ of the drug on a paper ruler applicator.
3. absorption
4. 2 suppositories
5. 2 suppositories
6. 1 suppository
7. 2 suppositories
8. 2 suppositories

Answers to review problems

1. a) Monistat-Derm cream
   b) miconazole nitrate
   c) 2% cream
2. When topical ointment is ordered for wound care, the amount to apply is left to the nurse's judgment.
3. The nurse should measure 1½″ of the drug on a paper ruler applicator.
4. 1 suppository
5. 2 suppositories
6. ½ suppository
7. ½ suppository
8. 1 suppository

UNIT 5

◆

Calculating Parenteral Dosages

Parenteral medications may be supplied as liquids or as powders that must be reconstituted. For both types of parenteral drugs, the nurse must be able to accurately calculate the amount of medication to administer. For drugs that require reconstitution, the nurse must also be able to calculate the amount of diluent to add to the powder.

Unit 5 prepares you to calculate and administer parenteral medications. Chapter 13 introduces the syringes, needles, and related calculations you may use for parenteral administration. Chapter 14 shows you how to read parenteral drug labels, providing many different examples. Chapter 15 discusses single- and multiple-strength powders and describes how to reconstitute them. It also describes how to handle prepared solutions. Chapter 16 highlights insulin administration. After reviewing diabetes and insulin therapy, it introduces insulin syringes and needles, explains how to read and process insulin orders, and demonstrates how to administer insulin safely.

Chapters 17 through 19 address I.V. therapy. They walk you step-by-step through calculations for I.V. flow rates, infusion times, and selected I.V. medication dosages. As in the earlier chapters, the skills in these chapters are vital. They help you ensure safe administration of parenteral medications and avoid errors that could harm the patient.

Chapter

13

◆

Syringes and Needles

To administer parenteral drugs safely, you must select and use the proper syringe and needle for the drug, its use, and the patient's condition. This chapter will show you how.

Hypodermic syringe measurements

The nurse may use three basic types of hypodermic syringes to measure and administer parenteral drugs: standard, tuberculin, and prefilled syringes. Although these syringes usually are calibrated in cubic centimeters (cc), the drugs they measure are ordered in milliliters (ml). Keep in mind that cc and ml are equivalents.

Standard syringes

Standard syringes are available in 3-, 5-, 10-, 20-, 30-, and 50-cc sizes. Each syringe consists of a plunger, barrel, hub, needle, and dead space. (See *Parts of a standard syringe* for an illustration.) The dead space holds the fluid that remains in the syringe and needle after the plunger is completely depressed. Some syringes, such as insulin syringes, do not have dead space. (See Chapter 16, Insulin Dosage Calculations, for details.)

Parts of a standard syringe

The illustration below identifies the key parts of a standard 3-cc syringe.

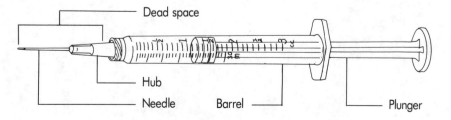

Dead space

Hub

Needle   Barrel   Plunger

Each standard syringe is calibrated in cubic centimeters. The most commonly used syringe is the 3-cc syringe. It is calibrated in tenths of a cc on the right and minims on the left; it includes larger marks for half a cc on the right. Larger-volume syringes are calibrated in two-tenths of a cc; they include larger marks for full cubic centimeters.

The nurse uses these calibrations to measure the drug. After calculating the dosage, the nurse draws up the drug into the syringe, using aseptic technique. The nurse pulls back the plunger until the top ring of the plunger's black portion aligns with the syringe calibration that represents the amount of the drug to be administered. Then, after double checking the drug measurement, the nurse administers the drug.

Tuberculin syringes

A tuberculin syringe holds up to 1 ml (or cc) of medication. Commonly used for intradermal injections, it is also used to administer a small volume of medication, such as to a pediatric or intensive-care patient. Each tuberculin syringe is calibrated in hundredths of a cc on the right and minims on the left, enabling the nurse to accurately administer a dose as small as 0.25 ml. Each syringe also has calibrations for alternate tenths of a cc: 0.20, 0.40, 0.60, and 0.80. (See *Parts of a tuberculin syringe* for an illustration.)

Parts of a tuberculin syringe

The illustration below identifies the key parts of a tuberculin syringe.

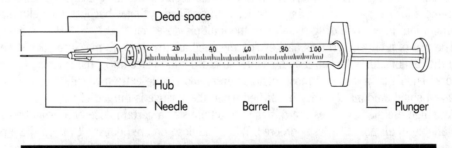

Measuring a drug with a tuberculin syringe is done the same as with a standard syringe. However, because the measurements on the tuberculin syringe are so small, the nurse must take extra care when reading the dose.

Prefilled syringes

A prefilled syringe is a sterile syringe filled with a premeasured dose of medication. It usually comes with a cartridge-needle unit and requires a special holder (Carpuject or Tubex) to release the medication from the cartridge. Each cartridge typically is calibrated in tenths of a milliliter and includes larger marks for half and full milliliters. (See *Parts of a prefilled syringe*, page 142, for an illustration.) Some cartridges allow for the addition of diluent or a second medication when a combined dose is ordered.

Parts of a prefilled syringe

The illustration below identifies the key parts of a prefilled syringe.

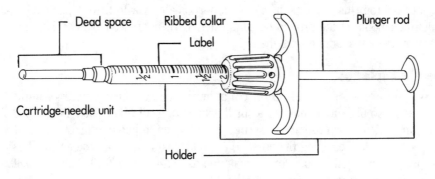

Prefilled syringes are labeled with the medication name and dose. This reduces preparation time and the risk of medication errors. Because this also simplifies recording the amount of drug used, narcotics commonly are supplied in prefilled syringes. When drugs are supplied in multiple-dose vials, instead of prefilled syringes, it is difficult to determine the amount of drug that remains in the vial. This interferes with accurate recording of drug usage, which is a legal requirement for narcotics. Recording is easier with prefilled syringes because they eliminate any guessing about how much drug remains in the multiple-dose vial.

The use of prefilled syringes also avoids the need for the nurse to measure each dose because the manufacturer has already measured the drug and placed it in the syringe. However, the nurse should be aware that most manufacturers add a little extra medication to the syringe because a small amount of it may be wasted when the syringe is purged of air.

Although prefilled syringes are designed to administer a certain dose of a drug, they are not available in all possible doses ordered. When the dose ordered does not match the amount in the prefilled syringe, the nurse must perform a dosage calculation to determine the amount of the drug needed. Then the nurse should discard the extra drug in the syringe by expelling it from the syringe. If the drug is a narcotic, the nurse must document the amount of the drug that was wasted. Another nurse must witness the expulsion of the drug and must cosign the narcotic record.

Closed-system device

A closed-system device is another type of prefilled syringe. It comes with the needle and syringe in place and a separate prefilled medication chamber. Emergency drugs, such as atropine and lidocaine, are available in these prefilled syringes.

To prepare a closed-system device, hold the medication chamber in one hand and the syringe and needle in the other. Flip the protective caps off both ends. Insert the medication chamber into the syringe section. Remove the needle cap and expel any air and any extra medication in the system.

Hypodermic syringe measurements

Answer the following questions about syringe measurements. To check your answers, see page 147.

1. Identify the dose contained in the standard syringe below.

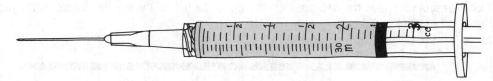

2. Identify the dose contained in the standard syringe below.

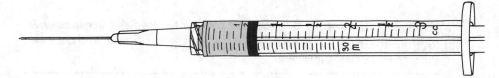

3. What is the first calibration on a 3-ml standard syringe?

4. Identify the dose contained in the tuberculin syringe below.

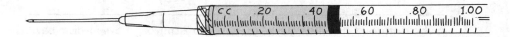

5. Identify the dose contained in the tuberculin syringe below.

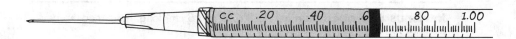

6. A pediatric patient needs 0.25 mg of a drug, which is supplied in a vial that reads 1 mg/ml. Which tuberculin syringe calibration corresponds to the dose the patient should receive?

7. The doctor prescribes 0.125 mg of a drug that comes in a vial containing 0.25 mg/ml. Which tuberculin syringe calibration corresponds to the dose the nurse should administer?

8. A patient must receive 0.26 mg of a drug but the drug is supplied in a form that provides 1 mg/ml. Which tuberculin syringe calibration corresponds to the dose the patient should receive?

9. A prefilled syringe contains a 50-mg dose in 2 ml and has a volume of 2.2 ml. Should the nurse administer the entire prefilled syringe to a patient who needs a 50-mg dose?

10. The nurse must add 0.6 ml of a drug to a prefilled syringe that contains 0.5 ml of a different drug. After the nurse does this, what is the total drug volume in the syringe?

11. To a prefilled syringe that contains 1 ml of a drug, the nurse adds 0.9 ml of a second drug. What is the total drug volume in the syringe?

Types and sizes of needles

When choosing a needle, the nurse must consider the needle gauge (G), bevel, and length. *Gauge* refers to the inside diameter of the needle. The smaller the gauge, the larger the diameter. For example, a 14G needle has a larger diameter than a 25G needle. *Bevel* refers to the angle at which the needle tip is opened. A needle's bevel may be considered short, medium, or long. *Length* describes the distance from the tip to the hub of the needle. Needle length ranges from ⅜″ to 3″ (1 to 7.5 cm).

Needle selection guide

When choosing a needle, the nurse must consider the needle's purpose as well as its gauge, bevel, and length. Use the following selection guide to choose the right needles for your patients.

Intradermal needles are ⅜″ to ⅝″ (1 to 1.5 cm) long, usually have short bevels, and are 25G in diameter.

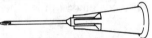

Subcutaneous needles are ½″ to ⅞″ (1.3 to 2 cm) long, have medium bevels, and are 25G to 23G in diameter.

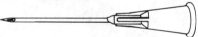

Intramuscular needles are 1″ to 3″ (2.5 to 7.5 cm) long, have medium bevels, and are 23G to 18G in diameter.

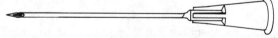

Intravenous needles are 1″ to 3″ long, have long bevels, and are 25G to 14G in diameter.

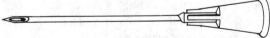

Filter needles, which should *not* be used for injection, are 1½″ (4 cm) long, have medium bevels, and are 20G in diameter. Microscopic pieces of rubber or glass may enter the solution when the nurse punctures the diaphragm of a vial with a needle or snaps open an ampule. The nurse can use a filter needle with a screening device in the hub to remove minute particles of foreign material from a solution.

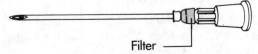

Filter

Different types of needles are designed for different purposes. The basic types of needles include intradermal, subcutaneous, intramuscular, intravenous, and filter needles. (See *Needle selection guide* for illustrations.)

Types and sizes of needles

Fill in the blanks in the following statements about needles. To check your answers, see page 147.

1. _____ refers to the inside diameter of a needle.

2. _____ refers to the angle at which the needle tip is opened.

3. The _____ the gauge, the _____ the diameter of a needle.

4. The needle's length is measured from the tip to the _____ of the needle.

5. The nurse should use a _____ needle to withdraw a solution from a glass ampule or a vial with a rubber stopper.

Calculations for drugs in syringes

At times, the nurse may need to calculate dosages of drugs that are administered by syringe. To do this, the nurse can use ratios or fractions in a proportion, as in this example.

◆ *A patient needs to receive 4 mg of a drug, and the vial contains 2 mg/ml. Which standard syringe calibration corresponds to the dose the patient should receive?*

◆ Set up a proportion with the known and unknown quantities.

$$\frac{4 \text{ mg}}{X} = \frac{2 \text{ mg}}{1 \text{ ml}}$$

◆ Solve for X.

$$X \times 2 \text{ mg} = 4 \text{ mg} \times 1 \text{ ml}$$

$$X = \frac{4 \text{ mg} \times 1 \text{ ml}}{2 \text{ mg}}$$

$$X = 2 \text{ ml}$$

◆ Consider the relationship of the dosage to the syringe.

The nurse should draw up 2 ml of the drug, which corresponds to the 2-cc calibration on a standard syringe.

Calculations for drugs in syringes

Perform the following calculations related to syringes. To check your answers, see page 147.

1. A doctor prescribes 50 mg of a drug for a patient but the drug is supplied in a vial marked 100 mg/ml. Which standard syringe calibration corresponds to the dose the nurse should administer?

2. A prefilled syringe is filled to the 2-ml mark and its label states that it contains 4 mg. The patient must receive 3 mg of the drug. How many milliliters should remain in the syringe for administration?

3. A prefilled syringe contains 15 mg of a drug and is filled to the 1-ml mark. If a patient requires 7 mg of the drug, how many milliliters should the nurse administer?

4. A standard 3-cc syringe is filled to the 0.8-cc mark with a drug from a vial that contains 50 mg/ml. What is the dose (in milligrams) contained in the syringe?

Review problems

Answer the following questions about syringes and needles. To check your answers, see page 148.

1. Which type of syringe is calibrated in hundredths and minims?

2. Which type of syringe commonly is used for narcotics because it simplifies recording of the amount of drug used?

3. Which type of syringe reduces preparation time and the risk of medication errors?

4. Which type of syringe includes no dead space?

5. To a prefilled syringe that contains 1 ml of a drug, the nurse adds 0.7 ml of a second drug. Now what is the total drug volume in the syringe?

6. To a prefilled syringe that contains 2 ml of a drug, the nurse adds 0.4 ml of a second drug. Now what is the total drug volume in the syringe?

7. A patient must receive 0.75 mg of a drug from a vial that contains 1 mg/ml. Which syringe calibration on a tuberculin syringe corresponds to the dose the patient should receive?

8. Using a tuberculin syringe, the nurse must administer 0.25 mg of a drug from a vial that contains 1 mg/ml. Which calibration corresponds to the dose the nurse should administer?

9. Tuberculin syringes commonly are used to administer what type of injections?

10. A prefilled syringe is filled to the 1.2-ml mark with a drug solution that contains 1 mg/ml. What should the nurse do before administering a 1-mg dose from this syringe?

11. Minim calibrations appear on which side of a standard syringe?

12. A patient needs to receive 30 mg of a drug from a vial that contains 10 mg/ml. Which syringe calibration on a standard syringe corresponds to the dose the patient should receive?

13. Emergency drugs usually are administered in which type of device?

14. Which type of needle should *not* be used for injection?

15. Which type of needle is ⅜″ to ⅝″ long and has a short bevel?

16. Which type of needle is 1″ to 3″ long and has a medium bevel?

17. Which type of needle is ½″ to ⅞″ long and 25G to 23G in diameter?

18. Which type of needle is 1″ to 3″ long, has a long bevel, and is 25G to 14G in diameter?

19. A standard 3-cc syringe is filled to the 1.2-cc mark with a drug from a vial marked 8 mg/ml. What is the dose (in milligrams) contained in the syringe?

20. A prefilled syringe is filled to the 1-cc mark, and its label states that it contains 8 mg. The patient must receive 6 mg of the drug. How many milliliters should the nurse administer?

21. A tuberculin syringe is filled to the 0.6 cc-mark with a drug from a vial marked 10 mg/ml. How many milligrams of the drug are contained in the syringe?

Answers to practice problems

♦ Hypodermic syringe measurements

1. 2½ or 2.5 ml
2. 0.6 ml
3. 0
4. 0.45 ml
5. 0.6 ml
6. 0.25 cc
7. 0.5 cc
8. 0.26 cc
9. No. Prefilled syringes contain extra solution for engaging the needle and expelling air before injection.
10. 1.1 ml
11. 1.9 ml

♦ Types and sizes of needles

1. Gauge
2. Bevel
3. smaller, larger
4. hub
5. filter

♦ Calculations for drugs in syringes

1. ½ cc
2. 1.5 ml
3. 0.47 ml
4. 40 mg

Answers to review problems

1. tuberculin syringe
2. prefilled syringe
3. prefilled syringe
4. insulin syringe
5. 1.7 ml
6. 2.4 ml
7. 0.75 cc
8. 0.25 cc
9. intradermal
10. The nurse should discard the extra 0.2 ml of solution; it is supplied to engage the needle before injection.
11. left side
12. 3 cc
13. closed-system device (a type of prefilled syringe)
14. filter needle
15. intradermal needle
16. intramuscular needle
17. subcutaneous needle
18. intravenous needle
19. 9.6 mg
20. 0.75 ml
21. 6 mg

Chapter

14

Parenteral Drugs and Labels

Before you can administer parenteral drugs, you must be familiar with these drugs and their labels. By reading and working through this chapter, you will become adept at reading parenteral drug labels, dealing with different types of solutions, measuring parenteral drugs, and performing basic dosage calculations for parenteral solutions.

Parenteral drugs are medications that must be administered by injection—usually by the intravenous (I.V.), intramuscular (I.M.), and subcutaneous (S.C.) routes. Manufacturers package parenteral drugs in glass ampules, single- or multiple-dose vials with rubber stoppers, and pre-filled syringes or cartridges. They manufacture parenteral drugs for the I.M. and S.C. routes in various dosage strengths (concentrations) so that the usual adult dose can be contained in 1 to 3 ml of solution. (If a patient needs a dose larger than 3 ml, the nurse should give it in two injections at two different sites to ensure proper drug absorption.)

Usually, you'll prepare I.V. medications in two steps. First, draw up the medication to obtain the correct dose. Then, dilute it further by drawing up another solution into the syringe or adding the medication to I.V. fluid.

Parenteral solution labels

Reading the label of a parenteral solution is much like reading the label of an oral solution. The label contains the solution's trade name (some manufacturers occasionally do not use a trade name because the generic name is so well known), followed by its generic name, the total volume of solution in the container, dosage strength or concentration (which for parenteral drugs is the drug dose present in a volume of solution), and expiration date. The label may also contain special instructions, such as *for I.V. administration only* (see the sample solution label below).

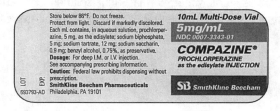

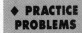

◆ **PRACTICE PROBLEMS**

Parenteral solution labels

Answer the following questions about reading solution labels. To check your answers, see page 157.

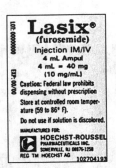

1. Based on the solution label above, answer these questions.
   a) What is the drug's trade name?
   b) What is the drug's generic name?
   c) What is the drug's dosage strength?
   d) What is the total drug volume in the container?
   e) By which routes can this drug be administered?

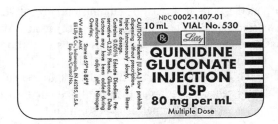

2. Based on the label above, answer these questions.
   a) What is the drug's trade name?
   b) What is the drug's generic name?
   c) What is the drug's dosage strength?
   d) What is the total drug volume in the container?
   e) By which routes can this drug be administered?

Percentage and ratio solutions

A *solution* is a liquid preparation that contains a *solute* (liquid or solid form of a drug) dissolved in a *diluent* (solvent), such as sterile water, normal saline solution, or dextrose 5% in water. Solutions come in different strengths (concentrations), which can be expressed as *percentage or ratio* solutions.

Percentage solutions

The clearest and most common way to label or describe a solution is as a percentage. This also is the easiest to use when making dosage calculations, dilutions, or alterations. A percentage solution may be expressed in terms of weight/volume (W/V) or volume/volume (V/V). In a W/V percentage solution, the percentage, or strength, refers to the number of grams of solute (weight) per 100 ml of finished solution (volume). In a V/V percentage solution, the percentage, or strength, refers to the number of milliliters of solute (volume) per 100 ml of finished solution (volume). This relationship can be expressed mathematically as:

% (W/V) = grams solute/100 ml finished solution

% (V/V) = milliliters solute/100 ml finished solution

This mathematical relationship lets the nurse know the contents of any percentage solution by reading its label, as shown in *Contents of percentage solutions.*

Contents of percentage solutions

The nurse can determine the contents of a weight/volume (W/V) or volume/volume (V/V) percentage solution by reading the label, as shown below.

PERCENTAGE SOLUTION	CONTENTS
5% (W/V) boric acid solution	5 g of boric acid in 100 ml of finished solution
0.9% (W/V) NaCl	0.9 g of sodium chloride in 100 ml of finished solution
5% (W/V) dextrose	5 g of dextrose in 100 ml of finished solution
2% (V/V) hydrogen peroxide	2 ml of hydrogen peroxide in 100 ml of finished solution
70% (V/V) isopropyl alcohol	70 ml of isopropyl alcohol in 100 ml of finished solution
10% (V/V) glycerin	10 ml of glycerin in 100 ml of finished solution

Ratio solutions

The strength of a ratio solution usually is expressed as two numbers separated by a colon. The first number in the ratio signifies the amount of a drug in grams (in a W/V solution) or in milliliters (in a V/V solution). The second number indicates the volume of finished solution in milliliters. This relationship can be expressed as:

ratio = amount of drug : amount of finished solution

See *Contents of ratio solutions* for more information.

Contents of ratio solutions

The nurse can determine the contents of a weight/volume (W/V) or volume/volume (V/V) ratio solution from the label, as shown below.

RATIO SOLUTION	CONTENTS
benzalkonium chloride 1:750	1 g of benzalkonium chloride in 750 ml of finished solution
silver nitrate 1:100	1 g of silver nitrate in 100 ml of finished solution
epinephrine (Adrenalin) 1:1,000	1 g of epinephrine in 1,000 ml of finished solution
Burow's solution (aluminum acetate) 1:40	1 g of aluminum acetate in 40 ml of finished solution

Any ratio solution can be converted to a percentage solution, using the proportion method. For example, to convert the Burow's solution in the chart to a percentage solution, use the ratio 1 g : 40 ml in a proportion with the unknown quantity and a finished solution of 100 ml.

$$1 \text{ g} : 40 \text{ ml} :: \text{X g} : 100 \text{ ml}$$

$$40 \text{ ml} \times \text{X g} = 1 \text{ g} \times 100 \text{ ml}$$

$$\text{X} = \frac{1 \text{ g} \times 100 \text{ ml}}{40 \text{ ml}}$$

$$\text{X} = 2.5 \text{ g}$$

$$\text{X} = 2.5\%$$

◆ **PRACTICE PROBLEMS**

Percentage and ratio solutions

Answer the following questions about percentage and ratio solutions. To check your answers, see page 157.

1. If a solution contains 1 g of epinephrine in 10,000 ml, what ratio should appear on the solution label?

2. If 100 ml of finished solution contains 25 g of mannitol, what percentage should appear on the solution label?

3. If a patient must receive 50 ml of 25% mannitol solution, how many grams will the patient receive?

4. The doctor prescribes one 50-ml vial of 50% dextrose solution. How many grams of dextrose does the vial contain?

5. In a 1-ml vial of epinephrine 1:1,000, what is the dosage strength of this solution?

Drugs measured in units

Some drugs, such as heparin, insulin, and penicillin G, are measured in units (U). The unit system measures drugs based on an international standard of drug potency—not on their weight. (See *Sample label of a drug measured in units* for an example. See *Uses and doses of heparin* for details about heparin. Also see Chapter 16, Insulin Dosage Calculations, for details about insulin.)

Sample label of a drug measured in units

As with other medications, the label of a parenteral drug measured in units must include the information shown below.

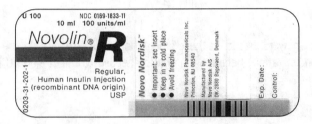

To perform dosage calculations for drugs measured in units, use the same guidelines as for calculations with other drugs, as shown in the following patient situation.

Uses and doses of heparin

The anticoagulant heparin is used in small doses to keep I.V. lines patent, in moderate doses to prevent thrombosis and embolism, and in large doses to treat these disorders. Because it is used in widely varying doses, heparin is commonly available in concentrations that range from 10 to 20,000 U/ml.

Before drawing up heparin or mixing it in I.V. solutions, the nurse should know what it will be used for, check all calculations for accuracy, and make sure that the heparin concentration is appropriate for the intended use. Dosage calculation errors with heparin can cause excessive bleeding or undertreatment of a clotting disorder.

A drug order calls for heparin 8,000 U S.C. q12h. Heparin is available in a 10,000 U/ml concentration and a 5,000 U/ml concentration. To determine which one would be best for S.C. administration, calculate the volumes for each strength.

◆ First, compute the volume for the 10,000 U/ml concentration, using the ratio and proportion method.

$$10,000 \text{ U} : 1 \text{ ml} :: 8,000 \text{ U} : X \text{ ml}$$

$$1 \text{ ml} \times 8,000 \text{ U} = 10,000 \text{ U} \times X \text{ ml}$$

$$\frac{1 \text{ ml} \times 8,000 \cancel{U}}{10,000 \cancel{U}} = X$$

$$0.8 \text{ ml} = X$$

◆ Then, compute the volume for the 5,000 U/ml concentration.

$$5,000 \text{ U} : 1 \text{ ml} :: 8,000 \text{ U} : X \text{ ml}$$

$$1 \text{ ml} \times 8,000 \text{ U} = 5,000 \text{ U} \times X \text{ ml}$$

$$\frac{1 \text{ ml} \times 8,000 \cancel{U}}{5,000 \cancel{U}} = X$$

$$1.6 \text{ ml} = X$$

◆ Compare the answers. Based on these calculations, the nurse would use the 10,000 U/ml dosage strength (concentration) because the volume needed to inject 8,000 U is smaller.

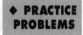

Drugs measured in units

Answer the following questions about drugs measured in units. To check your answers, see page 157.

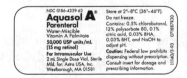

1. Based on the drug label above, answer these questions.

    a) What is the drug's dosage strength?

    b) What is the drug's generic name?

    c) What is the administration route for this drug?

    d) How many milliliters of the drug should the nurse draw up to administer a dose of 25,000 U?

    e) If 2.5 ml of the drug supplies the correct dose, then the dose contains how many units?

2. Answer the following questions based on this situation: Heparin sodium injection is available in a vial that contains 10,000 U/ml. This multiple-dose vial holds 4 ml of solution.

    a) If a patient must receive a dose of 5,000 U, how many milliliters of the drug should the nurse administer?

    b) If the doctor prescribes heparin sodium 25,000 U, how many milliliters of the drug should the nurse administer?

    c)   What is the drug's dosage strength?

    d)   If the nurse administers 1.25 ml of the drug, how many units does the patient receive?

    e)   How many units does this vial contain?

Drugs measured in milliequivalents

Electrolytes are measured in milliequivalents (mEq). Drug manufacturers provide information about the number of metric units required to provide the prescribed number of milliequivalents. For example, the manufacturer's instructions may indicate that 1 ml equals 4 mEq.

Patient situation

A patient needs 20 mEq of potassium chloride added to 1 L of I.V. fluids. The available vial of potassium chloride contains 2 mEq/ml. How many milliliters of potassium chloride must be added to the I.V. fluid?

◆ Set up the ratio.

$$2 \text{ mEq} : 1 \text{ ml} :: 20 \text{ mEq} : X \text{ ml}$$

◆ Solve for X.

$$2 \text{ mEq} \times X \text{ ml} = 1 \text{ ml} \times 20 \text{ mEq}$$

$$X \text{ ml} = \frac{20}{2}$$

$$X = 10 \text{ ml}$$

Ten milliliters of potassium chloride should be added to the I.V. fluid.

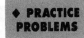

Drugs measured in milliequivalents

Answer the following questions about drugs measured in milliequivalents. To check your answers, see page 158.

1. A patient must receive 1 L of I.V. fluid with 40 mEq of potassium chloride added. The vial of potassium chloride solution contains 2 mEq/ml. How many milliliters should the nurse add to the I.V. fluid?

2. The doctor prescribes 8.5% sodium bicarbonate in a 35-mEq dose. If the drug vial contains 50 mEq/50 ml, how many milliliters should the patient receive?

3. The doctor orders 1 ampule of calcium gluconate for a patient. The nurse notes that a 10-ml ampule contains 0.465 mEq/ml. How many mEq of calcium gluconate should the patient receive?

4. A patient needs to receive sodium chloride injection 23.4% in a 30-mEq dose. The drug vial contains 4 mEq/ml. How many milliliters of solution should the nurse add to the patient's I.V. fluid?

5. A patient is to receive 1 L of I.V. fluid with 30 mEq of potassium chloride added. The vial contains 40 mEq of potassium chloride in a dosage strength of 2 mEq/ml. How many milliliters of potassium chloride solution should the nurse add to the I.V. fluid?

Review problems

Answer the following questions about parenteral drugs. To check your answers, see page 158.

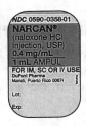

1. Based on the Narcan label above, answer these questions.
   a) What is the dosage strength?
   b) What is the administration route?
   c) If the doctor prescribes a 0.3-mg dose, how many milliliters of solution should the nurse administer?

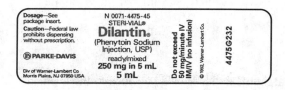

2. Based on the Dilantin label above, answer these questions.
   a) What is the total volume contained in the vial?
   b) What is the dosage strength?
   c) If a patient requires a 100-mg dose, how many milliliters of solution should the nurse administer?
   d) How many milligrams of Dilantin are contained in 3 ml of solution?

3. A patient must receive 25 ml of 25% mannitol solution. How many grams of mannitol does this dose contain?

4. In a 2% lidocaine solution, 1 ml contains how many milligrams?

5. Answer the following questions based on this information: A prefilled syringe contains epinephrine 1:10,000 solution.
   a) If a patient must receive 1 mg during resuscitation, how many milliliters of the drug will the nurse administer?
   b) What is the metric dose of the epinephrine contained in the prefilled syringe?

6. Answer the following questions based on this information: A 1-ml vial of heparin contains 5,000 U/ml.
   a) What is the drug's dosage strength?
   b) If the doctor prescribes 3,000 U, how many milliliters of the drug will the patient receive?
   c) How many vials will the nurse need to administer a 10,000-U dose?

7. A 20-ml vial of potassium chloride contains 40 mEq. How many milliequivalents of potassium chloride does each milliliter of solution contain?

8. A 50-ml vial of 8.5% sodium bicarbonate contains 50 mEq. How many milliequivalents of sodium bicarbonate does each milliliter contain?

9. A patient needs to receive 15 mEq of potassium chloride in 100 ml of I.V. fluid. The 20-ml vial contains 40 mEq of potassium chloride. How many milliliters should the nurse add to the I.V. fluid?

10. A 10-ml vial of calcium gluconate contains 0.465 mEq/ml. The doctor prescribes half a vial of the calcium gluconate solution. How many milliequivalents does half a vial contain?

Answers to practice problems

◆ *Parenteral solution labels*

1. a) Lasix
   b) furosemide
   c) 10 mg/ml or 40 mg/4 ml
   d) 4 ml
   e) I.M. and I.V.

2. a) none
   b) quinidine gluconate injection USP
   c) 80 mg/ml
   d) 10 ml
   e) I.V.

◆ *Percentage and ratio solutions*

1. 1:10,000
2. 25% mannitol
3. 12.5 g
4. 25 g
5. 1 mg/ml

◆ *Drugs measured in units*

1. a) 50,000 U/ml
   b) water-miscible vitamin A palmitate
   c) I.M.
   d) 0.5 ml
   e) 125,000 U

2. a) 0.5 ml
   b) 2.5 ml
   c) 10,000 U/ml
   d) 12,500 U
   e) 40,000 U

◆ **Drugs measured in milliequivalents**

1. 20 ml
2. 35 ml
3. 4.65 mEq
4. 7.5 ml
5. 15 ml

Answers to review problems

1. a) 0.4 mg/ml
   b) I.M., S.C., or I.V.
   c) 0.75 ml
2. a) 5 ml
   b) 250 mg/5 ml
   c) 2 ml
   d) 150 mg
3. 6.25 g
4. 20 mg/ml
5. a) 10 ml
   b) 1 mg/10 ml
6. a) 5,000 U/ml
   b) 0.6 ml
   c) 2 vials
7. 2 mEq
8. 1 mEq
9. 7.5 ml
10. 2.325 mEq

Chapter

15

Reconstitution and Use of Parenteral Drugs

Some drugs are manufactured and packaged as powders because they become unstable quickly when they are in solution. When the doctor prescribes such a drug, the nurse or pharmacist must reconstitute it before it can be administered. This chapter will show you how to reconstitute powders and perform drug-related calculations.

Reconstitution of powders

Powders come in single-strength or multiple-strength formulations. A single-strength powder may be reconstituted to only one dosage strength (per route of administration), which is specified by the manufacturer. A multiple-strength powder can be reconstituted to various dosage strengths by adjusting the amounts of diluent and powder. When reconstituting a multiple-strength powder, the nurse must check the drug label or package insert for the dosage-strength options and choose the one that is closest to the ordered dosage strength.

This section provides general guidelines for handling single-strength and multiple-strength powders. For specific details on multiple-strength powder, see "Special considerations in reconstitution."

If you must reconstitute a powder for parenteral use, keep the following points in mind.

♦ When reconstituting a powder for injection, consult the drug label. It should give the total quantity of drug in the vial or ampule, the amount and type of diluent to add to the powder, and the strength and shelf life (expiration date) of the resulting solution. When diluent is added to a powder, the powder increases the fluid volume. For this reason, the label calls for less diluent than the total volume of the prepared solution. For example, you may have to add 1.7 ml of diluent to a vial of powdered drug to obtain a 2-ml total volume of prepared solution. Follow the directions on the drug label.

♦ To determine how much solution to administer, use the manufacturer's information about the dosage strength (concentration) of the solution. For example, to administer 500 mg of a drug when the dosage strength of the prepared solution is 1 g (1,000 mg) per 10 ml, set up a proportion with fractions as follows.

$$\frac{X \text{ ml}}{500 \text{ mg}} = \frac{10 \text{ ml}}{1,000 \text{ mg}}$$

◆ Solve for X.

$$X \text{ ml} \times 1{,}000 \text{ mg} = 500 \text{ mg} \times 10 \text{ ml}$$

$$X = \frac{500 \text{ mg} \times 10 \text{ ml}}{1{,}000 \text{ mg}}$$

$$X = \frac{5{,}000 \text{ ml}}{1{,}000}$$

$$X = 5 \text{ ml}$$

Patient situations

The doctor prescribes 1.5 g of cefazolin (Ancef) for a patient. One-gram vials of powdered drug are available. The label states: **Add 4.5 ml sterile water to yield 1 g/5 ml. How many milliliters of reconstituted cefazolin should the nurse give the patient?**

◆ First, dilute the powder according to the instructions on the label. The dosage strength (concentration) listed on the label provides the first fraction for the proportion.

$$\frac{1 \text{ g}}{5 \text{ ml}}$$

◆ Next, set up a proportion with the dosage strength (concentration) and the unknown quantity. Make sure the same units of measure appear in both denominators of the proportion. In this case, the units must both be grams or milligrams.

$$\frac{X \text{ ml}}{1.5 \text{ g}} = \frac{5 \text{ ml}}{1 \text{ g}}$$

$$X = \frac{1.5 \text{ g} \times 5 \text{ ml}}{1 \text{ g}}$$

◆ Solve for X.

$$X \text{ ml} \times 1 \text{ g} = 1.5 \text{ g} \times 5 \text{ ml}$$

$$X = 7.5 \text{ ml}$$

7.5 ml of the solution will deliver 1.5 g of cefazolin.

A patient is to receive 25 mg of gentamicin I.M. The label states: **Add 1.3 ml sterile diluent to yield 50 mg/1.5 ml.** *How many milliliters of fluid should the nurse add to the powder? How many milliliters of the resultant solution should the patient receive?*

◆ First, determine the amount of diluent to add to the vial. Because the label indicates how many milliliters of diluent to add, simply add that quantity (1.3 ml).

Note: Because the label contains this information, you do not need to perform a calculation using the figures given for the resultant solution strength or the amount of medication ordered.

◆ Next, calculate the volume of injection for 25 mg, using ratios in a proportion.

$$50 \text{ mg} : 1.5 \text{ ml} :: 25 \text{ mg} : X \text{ ml}$$

$$1.5 \text{ ml} \times 25 \text{ mg} = 50 \text{ mg} \times X \text{ ml}$$

$$\frac{1.5 \text{ ml} \times 25}{50} = X$$

$$0.75 \text{ ml} = X$$

The patient should receive 0.75 ml of the gentamicin solution.

Two-chambered vial with rubber stopper

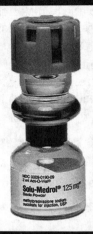

Some medications that require reconstitution are packaged in vials with two chambers separated by a rubber stopper. (See *Two-chambered vial with rubber stopper* for a photograph.) The upper chamber contains the diluent, and the lower chamber contains the powdered drug. When the nurse depresses the top of the vial, the rubber stopper between the two chambers dislodges, allowing the diluent to flow into the lower chamber, where it can mix with the powdered drug. Then the nurse can remove the correct amount of solution with a syringe.

◆ PRACTICE PROBLEMS

Reconstitution of powders

Answer the following questions about reconstitution. To check your answers, see page 166.

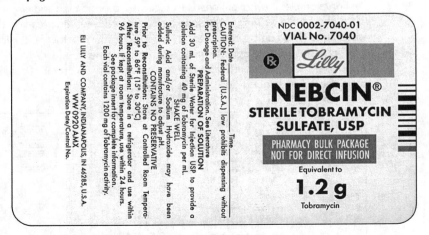

1. Based on the Nebcin label above, answer these questions.

a) Which diluent should the nurse use for reconstitution?

b) To obtain the correct dosage strength, the nurse should add how many milliliters of diluent?

    c)   What is the dosage strength of the reconstituted drug?

    d)   The doctor has prescribed an 80-mg dose of Nebcin for a patient. How many milliliters of solution should the nurse administer?

2.   A patient must receive Solu-Medrol 100 mg I.M. After reconstitution, the two-chambered vial contains a dosage strength of 125 mg/2 ml. How many milliliters of solution should the nurse administer?

3.   The doctor prescribes Solu-Cortef 200 mg I.V. for a patient. The nurse has a vial that, when reconstituted, contains a dosage strength of 500 mg/ 4 ml. How many milliliters of solution should the patient receive?

Special considerations in reconstitution

When the nurse reconstitutes a powder, two situations require special consideration: when the powder is available in multiple strengths and when the reconstitution information appears in the package insert instead of the drug label.

Multiple-strength powders

Some powdered drugs are available for reconstitution in multiple-strengths. When dealing with such a powder, the nurse must choose the most appropriate strength for the prescribed dose. (See *Sample multiple-strength powder.*)

Sample multiple-strength powder

Many drugs are available in more than one strength. For example, nafcillin sodium for injection comes in three dosage strengths (concentrations) — 20 mg/ml, 40 mg/ml, and 100 mg/ml — as shown below. The availability of multiple strengths allows the nurse to select the one that's most appropriate for the patient's needs.

    For example, if a patient needs to receive 1 g of nafcillin sodium, the nurse should choose the 100 mg/ml dosage strength because it requires less fluid to reconstitute. (This can be critical for a patient who must restrict fluid intake.) As the label states, this dosage strength requires the nurse to add 19 ml of diluent. Once the powder is reconstituted, the nurse can draw up 10 ml of solution to administer the prescribed dose of 1 g.

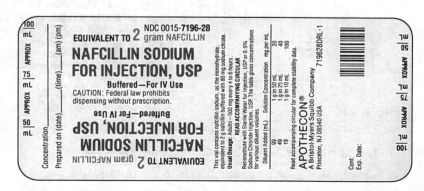

Reconstitution using package-insert information

When a drug's label supplies no information about reconstitution, the nurse must consult the package insert. The insert contains information on the type and amount of diluent needed, the dosage strength after reconstitution, and special information for administration and storage.

For example, the drug label for ceftazidime for injection provides no information about reconstitution, but refers the nurse to see the package insert for reconstitution instructions. So the nurse must read the package insert, which contains this information:

Vial size	Diluent to be added	Approximate available	Approximate average concentration
I.M. or I.V. direct (bolus) injection			
1 g	3.0 ml	3.6 ml	280 mg/ml
I.V. infusion			
1 g	10 ml	10.6 ml	95 mg/ml
2 g	10 ml	11.2 ml	180 mg/ml

The package insert also supplies special instructions for drawing up the drug and storing it, stating that the drug is good for 18 hours at room temperature or for 7 days if refrigerated.

Special considerations in reconstitution

Answer the following questions about reconstitution. To check your answers, see page 166.

1. Based on the label in *Sample multiple-strength powder,* answer these questions.

    a) What diluent is recommended for reconstitution?

    b) What is the total dose contained in this vial?

    c) To yield a dosage strength of 40 mg/ml, the nurse should add how much diluent?

    d) After the nurse adds sufficient diluent to yield a dosage strength of 40 mg/ml, what is the total volume of the vial?

    e) The doctor prescribes 500 mg of nafcillin sodium for I.M. injection. The nurse reconstitutes the drug to a dosage strength of 20 mg/ml. How many milliliters of the drug should the nurse administer?

2. Based on the following information, answer the questions below. A patient must receive 1,000,000 U of penicillin G potassium I.V. The drug label reads:

ml of diluent	U/ml of solution
20.0	50,000
10.0	100,000
4.0	250,000
1.8	500,000

a) If the nurse adds 1.8 ml of diluent to the vial, what is the dosage strength?

b) How many milliliters of the drug should the nurse draw up from the vial to administer the prescribed dose?

c) To reconstitute the drug to a dosage strength of 250,000 U/ml, how many milliliters of diluent should the nurse use?

3. The nurse should consult the _____ _____ if the drug label does not include reconstitution information.

4. Based on the ceftazidime package-insert chart on page 163, answer these questions.

a) The doctor prescribes ceftazidime 2 g by I.V. infusion. How much diluent should the nurse add to the vial?

b) The nurse adds sufficient diluent to provide a 2-g dose of ceftazidime. What is the total volume contained in the vial?

c) The nurse reconstituted ceftazidime at 1 A.M. on September 2 and stored it at room temperature. When will the solution expire?

5. Based on the ceftazidime package-insert chart on page 163, how many milliliters should the nurse draw up if the drug is reconstituted to a dosage strength of 95 mg/ml and the patient needs a 500-mg dose?

Handling prepared solutions

Besides including reconstitution information, the drug's label or package insert identifies the length of time the drug can be stored—usually under refrigeration and at room temperature—after reconstitution.

Once a drug is reconstituted, the nurse or pharmacist who prepared the solution must label it with the following information:

◆ preparer's initials
◆ reconstitution date
◆ expiration date
◆ dosage strength (if multiple-strength).

Handling prepared solutions

Answer the following questions about prepared solutions. To check your answers, see page 166.

1. A patient must receive Nebcin 100 mg I.V., which was reconstituted on September 15 at 9 A.M. When refrigerated, this solution expires 96 hours after reconstitution. What is the solution's expiration date?

2. The drug's label or package insert gives reconstitution information and identifies the length of time the drug can be _____ .

3. After reconstituting a multiple-strength solution, the nurse should label it with what information?

4. At 11 P.M. on June 5, the nurse reconstituted a drug and then stored it at room temperature. After reconstitution, its shelf life is 72 hours. When will the drug expire?

Review problems

Answer the following questions about parenteral drug reconstitution and use. To check your answers, see page 167.

1. A patient is to receive 3.1 g ticarcillin (Ticar) IVPB. The vial label states: *Add 18.5 ml of diluent for 0.155 g/ml solution.* How many milliliters should the nurse administer?

2. A patient must receive 1 g chloramphenicol (Cloromycetin) IVPB. The label states: *Add 10 ml of sterile aqueous diluent.* When reconstituted as directed, 10 ml contains the equivalent of 1 g chloramphenicol. If the powder is reconstituted as directed, what is the dosage strength (concentration) of the solution (in mg/ml)? How many milliliters of the solution should the patient receive?

3. A doctor prescribes metronidazole hydrochloride (Flagyl) 250 mg IVPB The vial states: *Add 4.4 ml of sterile diluent to provide an approximate volume of 5 ml.* The dosage strength is 100 mg/ml. How many milliliters of solution should the nurse draw up to administer the correct dose?

4. A patient needs to receive 75 mg of Solu-Medrol I.V. When reconstituted, the two-chambered vial contains 125 mg/2 ml. How many milliliters should the nurse administer?

5. The nurse reconstitutes Solu-Medrol as directed at 9 A.M. on May 26. The drug expires 48 hours after reconstitution. When does the Solu-Medrol expire?

6. A patient is to receive 500 mg cefazolin (Kefzol) IVPB. The vial label states: *1 g Kefzol, add 3 ml diluent for solution of 250 mg/ml.* How many milliliters should the nurse administer?

7. A doctor prescribes methicillin (Staphcillin) 2 g IVPB, and 1-g vials are available. A 1-g vial requires 5 ml of diluent to produce a 200 mg/ml solution. How many milliliters should the nurse administer?

8. A child is to receive 400 mg of ceftazidime (Fortaz) IVPB. The label states: *1 g Fortaz, add 10 ml diluent for 100 mg/ml solution.* How many milliliters should the nurse administer?

9. A child is to receive 1 g mezlocillin (Mezlin) IVPB. The label on a 2-g vial states: *Add 20 ml diluent for 100 mg/ml solution.* How many milliliters should the nurse administer?

10. A doctor prescribes ticarcillin (Ticar) 2 g IVPB q6h. The vial label states: *1 g Ticar. Add 2 ml diluent for 500 mg/ml solution.* How many milliliters should the nurse administer?

11. The patient must receive penicillin G potassium 600,000 U I.V. q4h. From the drug label of the multiple-strength powder, the nurse chooses a dosage strength of 200,000 U/ml. Then the nurse adds 4.6 ml of diluent as directed on the label. How many milliliters of the reconstituted drug should the nurse administer to the patient with each dose?

12. According to the label, penicillin G potassium expires 7 days after reconstitution, when refrigerated. The drug was reconstituted at 3 P.M. on May 22. When will the drug expire?

13. The doctor prescribes Claforan 1 g I.M. q8h. Following the package insert's reconstitution instructions, the nurse adds 3 ml of the appropriate diluent. The dosage strength of the reconstituted solution is 300 mg/ml. How many milliliters of the Claforan should the nurse administer with each dose?

14. When Claforan is stored at room temperature, it maintains its potency for 24 hours after reconstitution. The drug was reconstituted at 2 A.M. on January 31. When will it expire?

Answers to practice problems

◆ Reconstitution of powders

1. a) sterile water

b) 30 ml

c) 40 mg/ml

d) 2 ml

2. 1.6 ml

3. 1.6 ml

◆ Special considerations in reconstitution

1. a) sterile water or 0.9% sodium chloride injection

b) 2 g

c) 49 ml

d) 50 ml

e) 25 ml

2. a) 500,000 U/ml

b) 2 ml

c) 4 ml

3. package insert

4. a) 10 ml

b) 11.2 ml

c) September 2 at 7 P.M.

5. 5.3 ml

◆ Handling prepared solutions

1. September 19 at 9 A.M.

2. stored

3. initials, reconstitution date, expiration date, and dosage strength (concentration)

4. June 8 at 11 P.M.

Answers to review problems

1. 20 ml
2. The solution's concentration would be 100 mg/ml; the patient would receive 10 ml.
3. 2.5 ml
4. 1.2 ml
5. May 28 at 9 A.M.
6. 2 ml
7. 10 ml (The nurse would administer two 1-g vials each containing 5 ml.)
8. 4 ml
9. 10 ml
10. 4 ml (The nurse would administer two 1-g vials each containing 2 ml.)
11. 3 ml
12. May 29 at 3 P.M.
13. 3.3 ml
14. February 1 at 2 A.M.

Chapter

16

Insulin Dosage Calculations

To handle the special needs of diabetic patients, the nurse must understand the disease and the different types of insulin available. This chapter not only describes diabetes, but also provides a thorough understanding of insulin therapy. It discusses administration equipment and routes, shows how to read insulin orders, and demonstrates how to perform dosage calculations related to insulin administration.

Understanding diabetes and insulin therapy

Insulin, a potent hormone produced by the pancreas, regulates carbohydrate metabolism, which is reflected in blood glucose levels. An absolute or relative lack of insulin results in diabetes.

Two major types of diabetes exist: insulin-dependent diabetes mellitus (type I), which typically is diagnosed before age 20 and requires long-term insulin therapy, and non-insulin-dependent diabetes mellitus (type II), which typically is diagnosed after age 40 and can be controlled by diet therapy and oral hypoglycemic agents, although exogenous insulin may be used occasionally to stabilize blood glucose levels.

Some insulins are derived from bovine or porcine pancreas and differ from human insulin by only two amino acids. Others are identical to human insulin and are produced by enzymatic conversion of pork insulin or by recombinant DNA techniques. Regardless of product type, insulin dosages must be calculated and administered carefully. They must be administered parenterally: by the subcutaneous (S.C.) route for managing chronic diabetes and by the intravenous (I.V.) route for managing acute diabetic ketoacidosis. When regular insulin is added to a large-volume parenteral solution, some of it binds to the tubing and container. Sometimes albumin is added; albumin binds with the insulin and prevents it from binding elsewhere.

♦ **PRACTICE PROBLEMS**

Understanding diabetes and insulin therapy

Fill in the blanks to answer the following questions about diabetes and insulin therapy. To check your answers, see page 179.

1. Insulin is a potent hormone produced by the _____ .

2. Insulin regulates _____ metabolism, which is reflected in blood _____ levels.

Insulin labels

The many types of insulin are not all interchangeable. Fortunately, their labels provide the information the nurse needs to administer the correct type and concentration. Even so, all the labels require careful reading because they may contain confusingly similar information.

When reading insulin labels, remember that one kind of insulin, such as lente, may come in different types, but that these types are not interchangeable. For example, if the doctor orders lente human insulin zinc suspension, the nurse should not substitute lente insulin zinc suspension USP. Otherwise, a hypersensitive patient could develop a severe allergic reaction.

- Lente human insulin zinc suspension (semisynthetic)
- Lente insulin, insulin zinc suspension USP (beef)
- Lente purified pork insulin zinc suspension USP
- NPH human insulin isophane suspension (semisynthetic)
- NPH insulin, isophane insulin suspension USP (beef)
- NPH purified pork isophane insulin suspension USP
- 70% NPH, human insulin isophane suspension and 30% regular, human insulin injection (semisynthetic)
- Regular human insulin injection (semisynthetic) USP
- Regular insulin, insulin injection USP (pork)
- Regular purified pork insulin injection USP
- Semilente insulin, prompt insulin zinc suspension USP (beef)
- Semilente purified pork prompt insulin zinc suspension USP
- Ultralente insulin, extended insulin zinc suspension USP (beef)
- Ultralente purified beef extended insulin zinc suspension USP

3. _____ -_____ diabetes usually is diagnosed before age 20 and requires long-term insulin therapy.

4. _____ -_____ -_____ diabetes usually is diagnosed after age 40 and can be controlled by diet and oral hypoglycemic agents.

5. To manage acute diabetic ketoacidosis, insulin must be administered by the _____ route.

Using appropriate equipment

To administer insulin therapy properly, the nurse must select the appropriate insulin and syringe to meet the patient's needs.

Types of insulin

Several types of insulin are available. To prevent confusion when reading the labels of insulin vials, the nurse will need to know the following terms:

- *Regular crystalline insulin* is an insulin precipitated with zinc at a neutral pH. It is the only type of insulin that can be administered I.V.
- *PZI* refers to a protamine, zinc, and insulin solution.
- *NPH,* or isophane insulin suspension, is an insulin in crystalline form with protamine and zinc.
- *Extended insulin zinc suspension,* or ultralente, consists of large insulin crystals with a high zinc content in a sodium acetate-sodium chloride solution.
- *Prompt insulin zinc suspension,* or semilente, refers to a noncrystalline insulin precipitated at a high pH.
- *Insulin zinc suspension,* or lente, consists of 70% ultralente and 30% semilente.

For examples of labeling information on insulin vials, see *Insulin labels,* page 169.

The various insulin preparations have been modified by combination with larger insoluble protein molecules to slow absorption and prolong activity. Thus, they differ in onset, peak, and

Pharmacokinetics of insulins

Depending on its pharmacokinetic properties, an insulin preparation may be rapid-acting, intermediate-acting, or long-acting, as shown in the table below.

DRUG	ONSET	PEAK	DURATION
Rapid acting			
prompt insulin zinc suspension (semilente)	½ to 1½ hr	5 to 10 hr	12 to 16 hr
regular insulin	½ to 1 hr	2 to 4 hr	6 to 8 hr
Intermediate acting			
insulin zinc suspension (lente)	1 to 2½ hr	7 to 15 hr	22 to 26 hr
isophane insulin suspension (NPH)	1 to 1½ hr	8 to 12 hr	18 to 24 hr
Long acting			
extended insulin zinc suspension (ultralente)	4 to 8 hr	10 to 30 hr	> 36 hr
protamine zinc insulin suspension (PZI)	4 to 8 hr	14 to 20 hr	36 hr

duration of action. (See *Pharmacokinetics of insulins* for a summary of these differences.) Because of these differences, insulins are classified as rapid-acting, intermediate-acting, and long-acting.

Insulin dosages, expressed in units (U) based on bioassay of activity, are available in three concentrations. U-100 (100 U of insulin per milliliter) is the most commonly used, "universal" concentration. U-40 (40 U of insulin per milliliter), a weaker solution, may be used by older patients. Another concentration, U-500 (500 U of insulin per milliliter), is available for the rare instances in which a patient needs an exceptionally large dose.

Types of syringes

The nurse must select the insulin syringe that is compatible with the strength (or concentration) of the insulin to be administered. For example, U-100 insulin requires a U-100 syringe, U-40 insulin requires a U-40 syringe, and U-500 insulin requires a U-500 syringe. The U-100 syringe is calibrated so that 1 ml holds 100 units of insulin. The U-40 syringe is calibrated so that 1 ml holds 40 units of insulin, and so on. A low-dose syringe also is an option for some patients. This U-100 syringe is designed to hold only 50 units of insulin or less.

Thus, if the doctor prescribes 20 U of U-100 regular insulin, the nurse should use a U-100 syringe and draw up the insulin to the 20-U mark. (See *Insulin syringes* for examples of the most common types.)

Insulin syringes

Several different syringes labeled in units are available for insulin administration. The examples below show a U-100 syringe, which can deliver up to 100 U of insulin, and a low-dose syringe, which can deliver up to 50 U of U-100 insulin. Low-dose syringes measure small doses of insulin and display calibrations in large numbers, which is helpful for diabetic patients with vision problems.

U-100

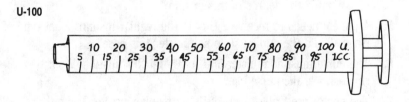

LOW-DOSE

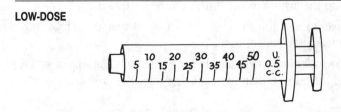

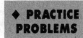

Using appropriate equipment

Answer the following questions about equipment for insulin therapy. To check your answers, see page 179.

1. Which type of insulin can be administered by the I.V. route?

2. What are the three classifications of insulin?

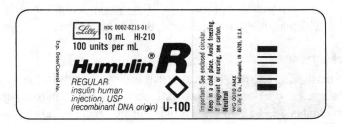

3. Based on the Humulin R label above, answer these questions.
   a) What type of insulin is Humulin R?
   b) What is its dosage strength?
   c) What is the source of this insulin?

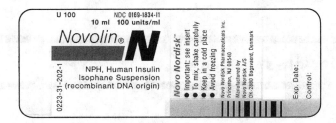

4. Based on the Novolin N label above, answer these questions.
   a) What type of insulin is Novolin N?
   b) What is its dosage strength?
   c) What is the source of this insulin?

5. A patient needs to receive 8 U of U-100 regular insulin. What type of syringe should the nurse use to administer this dose?

6. The nurse must administer 54 U of U-100 NPH insulin. What type of syringe should the nurse use?

7. The doctor prescribes 15 U of U-100 regular insulin. The nurse should draw up the insulin to what mark on the U-100 syringe?

8. A patient must self-inject U-40 insulin. What type of syringe should the nurse teach the patient to use?

9. The doctor orders U-500 insulin for a patient. What type of syringe should the nurse obtain to administer this type of insulin?

Reading insulin orders

When diabetes is diagnosed, the doctor orders blood and urine glucose determinations, usually in a hospital where the patient's diet is controlled, around-the-clock values can be measured, and blood and urine glucose baselines can be established. Based on these determinations, the doctor may order small doses of rapid-acting insulin at set times, such as every 4 hours or before meals and at bedtime, for several days. After a stable 24-hour dosage has been determined, the doctor may order dosage adjustments, such as one or two daily doses of intermediate-acting insulin, possibly accompanied by small doses of rapid-acting insulin.

For a newly diagnosed, ill, or unstable diabetic patient, the doctor may write an order on a sliding scale, which individualizes the insulin quantities and administration times according to the patient's age, exercise and work habits, desired degree of blood glucose level control, and response to insulin preparations, as shown in this example:

Blood glucose values	Insulin dose
< 180 mg/dl	No insulin
180 to 240 mg/dl	10 U of regular insulin S.C.
241 to 400 mg/dl	20 U of regular insulin S.C.
> 400 mg/dl	Call doctor for orders

Some patients may receive insulin doses based on home monitoring of blood glucose values with glucometers. In the past, patients also had their insulin doses adjusted on a sliding scale based on urine glucose values, as shown in this example:

Urine glucose values	Insulin dose
0 to ¼%	No insulin
½%	10 U of regular insulin
1%	15 U of regular insulin
2%	20 U of regular insulin

Such a patient might receive additional insulin if ketones appear in the urine.

When reading insulin orders, be alert to the placement of decimal points. Some patients are extremely sensitive to insulin, requiring a dose of less than 10 U. To clarify this, a doctor may write the dose with a decimal point, which may be overlooked on a line of writing and mistakenly dropped during transcription. For example, a doctor may want to prescribe 3 U of insulin and may write 3.0 U of insulin for clarity. If the decimal point is lost in transcription, the patient could receive 30 U of insulin, a tenfold dosing error. Always check doses that seem unusually large or small.

If an insulin order does not include the dosage strength, the nurse should administer U-100 insulin, which is known as the "universal" strength. If U-40 or U-500 insulin is required, it must be specified on the order.

Reading insulin orders

Answer the following questions about reading insulin orders. To check your answers, see page 179.

1. Based on the sliding scales above, answer these questions.
   a) If the patient's blood glucose level is 238 mg/dl, how many units of insulin should the patient receive?
   b) If the patient's blood glucose level is 169 mg/dl, how many units of insulin should the nurse administer?
   c) If the patient's urine glucose level is 1%, how many units of insulin should the patient receive?
   d) If the patient's blood glucose level is 435 mg/dl, how many units of insulin should the nurse administer?

2. A patient must receive 6 U of regular insulin S.C. To administer this dose, the nurse should draw up insulin to which mark on a U-100 syringe?

Processing insulin orders

Once insulin has been ordered, the nurse needs to draw it up and administer it. To ensure that the correct dose of the proper insulin is administered, follow this procedure:

• Read the vial label carefully, noting the type, concentration, source, and expiration date of the insulin. Most patients receive U-100 insulin, which contains 100 U of insulin per milliliter of solution or suspension. Others may receive U-40 insulin, which is used for patients accustomed to this concentration or those who need small doses, or U-500 insulin, which is used for patients with insulin resistance who require high doses.

• For regular crystalline insulin, ensure that it is clear and contains no particles. Discard any cloudy insulin or insulin with particles. Check that the storage conditions are appropriate and that the expiration date has not passed.

• Roll an insulin suspension between the palms of your hands to mix it properly. This is especially important when working with intermediate-acting insulins, which develop a sediment when standing.

   Do not shake the insulin. Shaking will create bubbles that mix air with the protein, which may disrupt its integrity and take up space in the syringe, causing an error in the insulin dose.

• Choose the appropriate syringe. Insulin syringes are designed to measure insulin accurately. When administering U-100 insulin, use a U-100 syringe, which is calibrated to measure up to 1 ml (100 U) of insulin in 1- or 2-U increments. When drawing up doses of less than 50 U, use a low-dose U-100 syringe, which is calibrated in 1-U increments. This type of syringe is particularly useful for drawing up doses of less than 20 U and may be easier to read for a diabetic patient with impaired vision.

• Clean the top of the vial with an alcohol swab.

• Insert the needle through the rubber diaphragm. Inject an amount of air into the vial equal to the amount of insulin to be withdrawn. Then invert or tilt the vial and withdraw the ordered amount of insulin into the syringe.

• Remove the syringe and needle from the vial.

• Recheck the insulin order and administer the medication.

Combining insulins

NPH and regular insulin commonly are administered concomitantly. When processing an order for this combination of drugs, draw them up into the same syringe following this procedure:

• Read the insulin order carefully.

• Read the vial labels carefully, noting the type, concentration, source, and expiration date of the drugs.

• Roll the NPH vial between the palms of your hands to mix it properly.

• Choose the appropriate syringe.

• Clean the tops of both vials with alcohol swabs.

• Inject air into the NPH vial equal to the amount of insulin you need to administer. Withdraw the needle and syringe, but do not withdraw any NPH insulin.

Golden Rules

When combining insulins, always draw up regular insulin *first* to avoid contamination with a longer-acting insulin.

- Now inject into the regular insulin vial an amount of air equal to the dose of regular insulin. Then invert or tilt the vial and withdraw the prescribed amount of regular insulin into the syringe. (Regular insulin is drawn up first to avoid contamination by the addition of longer-acting insulin.)
- Clean the top of the NPH vial again. Then insert the needle of the syringe containing the regular insulin into this vial and withdraw the prescribed amount of the NPH insulin.
- Mix the insulins in the syringe by pulling back slightly on the plunger and tilting the syringe back and forth.
- Recheck the drug orders, and administer the medications immediately.

Measuring insulin without an insulin syringe

If the only syringe available is calibrated in minims or milliliters, calculate the correct quantity using the proportion method (with ratios or fractions) or the desired-over-have method:

$$\frac{\text{desired amount of drug}}{\text{strength on hand}} = \frac{\text{unknown volume required (X)}}{\text{known volume of drug}}$$

Patient situations

A doctor prescribes 20 U of U-100 regular insulin. The only syringe on hand is a 1-ml tuberculin syringe. How many milliliters should the nurse administer?

♦ Set up a desired-over-have proportion with the known and unknown quantities.

$$\frac{20\ U}{100\ U} = \frac{X\ ml}{1\ ml}$$

♦ Solve for X.

$$100\ U \times X\ ml = 20\ U \times 1\ ml$$

$$X = \frac{20\ \cancel{U} \times 1\ ml}{100\ \cancel{U}}$$

$$X = 0.2\ ml$$

Administer 0.2 ml of U-100 regular insulin.

A patient is to receive 60 U of U-100 NPH insulin. No insulin syringes are available, so the nurse must determine how many milliliters to administer via a 1-ml syringe.

♦ Set up a proportion with the known and unknown quantities.

$$60\ U : X\ ml :: 100\ U : 1\ ml$$

◆ Solve for X.

$$X \text{ ml} \times 100 \text{ U} = 60 \text{ U} \times 1 \text{ ml}$$

$$X = \frac{60 \text{ U} \times 1 \text{ ml}}{100 \text{ U}}$$

$$X = 0.6 \text{ ml}$$

Administer 0.6 ml of U-100 NPH insulin.

The doctor prescribes 25 U of U-100 regular insulin. The only syringe available is a tuberculin syringe. How many milliliters of insulin should the nurse administer?

◆ Set up a proportion using the desired-over-have approach.

$$\frac{25 \text{ U}}{100 \text{ U}} = \frac{X \text{ ml}}{1 \text{ ml}}$$

◆ Solve for X.

$$100 \text{ U} \times X \text{ ml} = 25 \text{ U} \times 1 \text{ ml}$$

$$X = \frac{25 \text{ U} \times 1 \text{ ml}}{100 \text{ U}}$$

$$X = 0.25 \text{ ml}$$

The nurse will administer 0.25 ml of U-100 regular insulin.

Using insulin pumps and infusions

Close control of diabetes may delay the progression of some complications, such as renal impairment and retinopathy. Therefore, follow the therapeutic regimens carefully and administer insulin doses at the proper times. Be aware that some patients may receive continuous or intermittent S.C. infusions of insulin by small-infusion pumps. This method of drug delivery more closely mimics the body's normal pattern of insulin production. Other patients may receive insulin by the intranasal route. (For more information, see *Insulin infusion pumps.*)

Insulin infusion pumps

In most people, the pancreas normally secretes appropriate amounts of insulin in response to blood glucose levels. However, in patients with type I (insulin-dependent) diabetes, the pancreas cannot provide sufficient insulin to metabolize glucose. These patients need supplemental insulin. Although insulin usually is administered by subcutaneous injection, this route gives the patient little flexibility in mealtime or activity level because of the risk of hypoglycemia.

That is why many patients are beginning to receive supplemental insulin via an insulin pump, a programmable device that is inserted into the abdominal wall. Like the pancreas, the pump provides insulin in a continuous flow as well as in boluses at mealtimes, supplying the body with the exact amount of insulin it needs at the right time. The pump allows better control of the blood glucose level, which can prevent or slow the progress of complications of diabetes.

Patients with diabetic ketoacidosis may require a continuous I.V. infusion of regular insulin. The I.V. route is used because it allows rapid reduction of the blood glucose level, which the S.C. route cannot. (For more information, see Chapter 19, Specialized I.V. Medication Calculations.)

◆ **PRACTICE PROBLEMS**

Processing insulin orders

Answer the following questions about processing insulin orders. To check your answers, see pages 179 and 180.

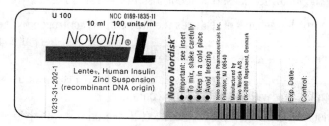

1. Based on the Novolin L label above, answer these questions.
   a) What type of insulin is Novolin L?
   b) What is its dosage strength?
   c) What type of syringe should the nurse obtain to administer this insulin?
   d) Before drawing up this insulin, what should the nurse do to mix it properly?
2. How should regular insulin look before administration?
3. A patient needs to receive 8 U of regular insulin and 25 U of NPH insulin. After the nurse combines the insulins, how many total units should the syringe contain?
4. The doctor prescribes 7 U of regular insulin and 32 U of NPH insulin for a patient. How many total units should the nurse draw up in the syringe?
5. A patient's daily insulin dose is 15 U of regular insulin and 22 U of lente insulin. How many total units of insulin does the patient receive?
6. A patient must receive a dose of 18 U of ultralente insulin and 4 U of regular insulin. What size syringe should the nurse use to administer this dose?
7. A patient needs to receive 10 U of U-100 regular insulin, but no insulin syringes are available. How many milliliters should the nurse administer in a 1-ml syringe?
8. The doctor prescribes 46 U of U-100 NPH insulin for a patient. If no insulin syringes are available, how many milliliters should the nurse administer in a 1-ml syringe?
9. The doctor prescribes 43 U of U-100 NPH insulin for a patient. The only syringe on hand is a tuberculin syringe. How many milliliters should the nurse administer?
10. A patient with _____ _____ may need continuous insulin infusion to rapidly reduce blood glucose levels.

11. Insulin infusion pumps closely mimic the body's normal pattern of insulin production. This helps delay the progression of _____ associated with diabetes.

Review problems

Answer the following questions about insulin therapy. To check your answers, see page 180.

1. Non-insulin-dependent diabetes mellitus can be controlled by diet therapy and _____ _____ _____ , although exogenous insulin may sometimes be required to stabilize blood glucose levels.

2. _____ is sometimes added to regular insulin infusions to prevent the insulin from binding with the tubing and container.

3. A doctor's order states: *30 U NPH S.C.* Based on this information, the nurse would draw up 30 U of _____ in a _____ syringe.

4. A doctor's order states: *60 U regular beef insulin S.C.* Based on this information, the nurse would draw up _____ insulin in a _____ syringe.

5. A doctor's order states: *15 U regular human insulin plus 40 U NPH human insulin S.C.* Based on this information, the nurse would use U-100 insulin. Which type of syringe should the nurse use? Which insulin should be drawn up first?

6. Based on the following sliding scale order, how many units of insulin should the nurse give to a patient whose most recent blood glucose level is 300 mg/dl?

Blood glucose values	Insulin dose
< 180 mg/dl	No insulin
180 to 250 mg/dl	10 U regular insulin S.C.
251 to 390 mg/dl	20 U regular insulin S.C.
> 390 mg/dl	Call doctor for orders

7. Which type of syringe should a nurse use to draw up U-100 insulin?

8. A doctor's order states: *Add 100 U of regular insulin to 500 ml of 0.45% sodium chloride, and infuse at 10 U/hr.* Which type of syringe would the nurse use to draw up the 100 U of regular insulin?

9. The nurse must administer 60 U of U-100 NPH insulin. No U-100 insulin syringes are available, so the nurse must use a 1-ml tuberculin syringe. How many milliliters of insulin should the nurse administer?

10. The doctor prescribes 30 U of NPH insulin and 6 U of regular insulin for a patient. No insulin syringes are available, but a 1-ml tuberculin syringe is. How many milliliters of insulin should the nurse administer?

11. What type of syringe should the nurse use to administer 4 U of U-100 insulin?

12. What should the nurse do if sediment appears in a vial of regular insulin?

13. Insulin infusion pumps can deliver intermittent or _____ S.C. infusions of insulin.

Answers to practice problems

◆ *Understanding diabetes and insulin therapy*

1. pancreas
2. carbohydrate, glucose
3. Insulin-dependent
4. Non-insulin-dependent
5. I.V.

◆ *Using appropriate equipment*

1. regular crystalline insulin
2. rapid-acting, intermediate-acting, and long-acting
3. a) regular
   b) 100 U/ml
   c) human
4. a) NPH
   b) 100 U/ml
   c) human
5. low-dose syringe
6. U-100 syringe
7. 15-U mark
8. U-40 syringe
9. U-500 syringe

◆ *Reading insulin orders*

1. a) 10 U of regular insulin
   b) No insulin should be administered.
   c) 15 U of regular insulin
   d) The nurse should call the doctor to determine the insulin dose.
2. 6-U mark

◆ *Processing insulin orders*

1. a) lente
   b) 100 U/ml
   c) U-100
   d) Roll the vial between the palms of the hands.
2. Regular insulin should look clear and should contain no particles.
3. 33 U
4. 39 U
5. 37 U
6. low-dose insulin syringe

7. 0.1 ml
8. 0.46 ml
9. 0.43 ml
10. diabetic ketoacidosis
11. complications

Answers to review problems

1. oral hypoglycemic agents
2. Albumin
3. NPH insulin 100 U/ml (U-100); U-100
4. 60 U of regular beef insulin (U-100); U-100
5. The nurse should use a U-100 syringe and draw up the regular insulin first.
6. 20 U
7. U-100 syringe
8. U-100 syringe
9. 0.6 ml
10. 0.36 ml
11. low-dose insulin syringe
12. The nurse should discard the vial because regular insulin should be clear.
13. continuous

Chapter

17

I.V. Flow Rate Calculations

Administering intravenous (I.V.) fluid safely is an important nursing skill, especially when you are caring for patients who are susceptible to fluid volume changes. To help you perfect this skill, Chapter 17 presents various methods for calculating flow rates accurately, describes how to regulate infusions manually and electronically, and demonstrates how to adjust the infusion rate as needed.

Identifying I.V. drip factors

To calculate the drip rate (number of drops to infuse per minute) of an I.V. solution, the nurse must first determine the drip factor (number of drops per milliliter of solution). The drip factor depends on the administration set to be used and is listed on the set's product label.

For a standard administration (macrodrip) set, the drip factor typically is 10, 15, or 20 gtt/ml; for a microdrip (minidrip) set, it is 60 gtt/ml. (See *I.V. drip rates,* page 182, for drip factors and drip rates of selected administration sets.)

Several factors influence the nurse's choice of administration set. For example, if a small volume must be infused, the nurse should use a microdrip set because it is easier to use and allows more accurate titration. (See *Determining which type of I.V. tubing to use,* page 183, for details.)

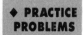

◆ PRACTICE PROBLEMS

Identifying I.V. drip factors

Answer the following questions about I.V. drip factors. To check your answers, see page 198.

1. What term describes the number of drops infused per minute?
2. What term describes the number of drops contained in 1 ml of I.V. fluid?
3. Based on *I.V drip rates,* page 182, answer these questions.
   a) The nurse must administer 1,000 ml of I.V. fluid over 8 hours. The tubing on hand is manufactured by Abbott. What is the drip factor?
   b) The nurse must administer 1,000 ml of I.V. fluid over 6 hours. The drip rate is 56 gtt/minute. What is the drip factor?

I.V. drip rates

When calculating the drip rate of I.V. solutions, remember that the number of drops required to deliver 1 ml varies with the type of administration set used and the manufacturer.

To calculate the drip rate, the nurse must know the drip factor for each manufacturer's product. As a quick guide, use the chart below.

MANUFACTURER	DRIP FACTOR	DROPS/MINUTE TO INFUSE (DRIP RATE)					
		500 ml/ 24 hr	1,000 ml/ 24 hr	1,000 ml/ 20 hr	1,000 ml/ 10 hr	1,000 ml/ 8 hr	1,000 ml/ 6 hr
		21 ml/hr	42 ml/hr	50 ml/hr	100 ml/hr	125 ml/hr	166 ml/hr
Abbott	15 gtt/ml	5 gtt	10 gtt	12 gtt	25 gtt	31 gtt	42 gtt
Baxter-Healthcare	10 gtt/ml	3 gtt	7 gtt	8 gtt	17 gtt	21 gtt	28 gtt
Cutter	20 gtt/ml	7 gtt	14 gtt	17 gtt	34 gtt	42 gtt	56 gtt
IVAC	20 gtt/ml	7 gtt	14 gtt	17 gtt	34 gtt	42 gtt	56 gtt
McGaw	15 gtt/ml	5 gtt	10 gtt	12 gtt	25 gtt	31 gtt	42 gtt

c) A patient needs to receive 1,000 ml of I.V. fluid over 10 hours. The drip rate is 17 gtt/minute. What is the drip factor?

d) The doctor prescribes 1,000 ml of I.V. fluid to run over 20 hours. The drip factor of the available tubing is 15 gtt/ml. What is the drip rate of this I.V. infusion?

Using the formula method

Doctors' orders for I.V. fluids or blood products usually specify a certain volume of fluid to be given over a particular length of time. By using this information and the drip factor in formulas, the nurse can calculate the flow rate and drip rate. Such calculations are said to use the formula method.

Flow rates

For patients receiving large-volume infusions (fluids given to maintain hydration or to replace fluids or electrolytes), the nurse may have to calculate the flow rate (the number of milliliters of fluid to administer over 1 hour) from the order, which may indicate the amount to administer

Determining which type of I.V. tubing to use

Most health care facilities stock I.V. tubing in several sizes. Microdrip (minidrip) tubing delivers 60 gtt/ml, and standard, or macrodrip, tubing delivers 10, 15, or 20 gtt/ml, depending on the manufacturer.

The rate and purpose of the infusion determine whether microdrip or macrodrip tubing should be used. For example, if a patient is to receive a solution at a rate of 125 ml/hour, macrodrip tubing is preferred. If microdrip tubing were used in this instance, the drip rate would be 125 gtt/minute, which is difficult to assess. Conversely, if a patient is to receive a solution at a rate of 10 ml/hour, microdrip tubing is preferred. If macrodrip tubing with a drip factor of 15 gtt/ml were used, the drip rate would be 3 gtt/minute. Maintaining I.V. patency at this rate is nearly impossible.

A rule of thumb for selecting I.V. tubing is to use macrodrip for any infusion with a rate of at least 80 ml/hour and microdrip for any infusion with a rate of less than 80 ml/hour or for a pediatric patient (to prevent fluid overload). Follow your facility's protocols.

When I.V. controllers and pumps are used, select the tubing specifically manufactured to work with that pump.

---

over 8 hours, 12 hours, or 24 hours. The calculations will depend on how the original orders were written and the facility's requirements for large-volume infusions. The calculations also can vary, depending on whether the volume ordered is per hour, per shift, or per day.

The flow rate can be determined with the following formula.

$$\text{Flow rate} = \frac{\text{total ml ordered}}{\text{specified number of hours}}$$

For example, if the patient is to receive 1,000 ml over 8 hours, the equation would be:

$$\text{Flow rate} = \frac{1,000 \text{ ml}}{8 \text{ hr}}$$

In this example, the flow rate would be 125 ml/hr. The nurse also will use the flow rate when working with I.V. infusion pumps to set the number of milliliters to be delivered in 1 minute. In that case, the flow rate would be divided by 60 minutes. This fraction would be:

$$\text{Rate per minute} = \frac{125 \text{ ml/hr}}{60 \text{ min}}$$

The infusion rate for 1 minute would be 2.08 ml/min, which can be rounded to 2 ml/min.

Drip rates

The nurse can use the following formula to determine the drip rate of an I.V. solution.

$$\text{Drip rate} = \frac{\text{total milliliters}}{\text{total minutes}} \times \text{drip factor}$$

First, set up a fraction showing the volume of the infusion over the number of minutes in which the volume is to be infused. For example, if a patient is to receive 200 ml of solution in 1 hour, the fraction would be:

$$\frac{200 \text{ ml}}{60 \text{ min}}$$

Next, multiply the fraction by the drip factor (the number of drops contained in 1 ml) to determine the number of drops per minute to be infused—the drip rate. Remember, the drip factor varies with the administration set and appears on the packaging containing the administration set. If, for example, the Abbott administration set were used, the drip factor would be 15 gtt/ml. The equation would be:

$$X = \frac{200 \text{ ml}}{60 \text{ min}} \times \frac{15 \text{ gtt}}{1 \text{ ml}}$$

$$X = \frac{3,000 \text{ gtt}}{60 \text{ min}}$$

$$X = 50 \text{ gtt/min}$$

The drip rate for this solution would be 50 gtt/min.

In practice, the drip rate may be observed for 15 seconds—sufficient time to determine whether the rate needs to be adjusted. To calculate the drip rate for 15 seconds, divide the drip rate per minute by 4. In the example, the equation would be:

$$\text{drip rate for 15 sec} = \frac{50 \text{ gtt/min}}{4}$$

In this example, the drip rate is 12.5 gtt/15 sec, rounded up to 13 gtt/15 sec. The nurse then would observe the drip chamber for 15 seconds to ensure that 13 drops are delivered.

Patient situations

A doctor's order calls for 1,000 ml of D$_5$W to be infused over 12 hours. Determine the drip rate for an administration set that delivers 15 gtt/ml.

◆ Set up the equation for determining the drip rate, and multiply the number of hours by 60 minutes in the denominator of the fraction.

$$X = \frac{1,000 \text{ ml}}{12 \text{ hr} \times 60 \text{ min}} \times 15 \text{ gtt/ml}$$

$$X = \frac{1,000 \text{ ml}}{720 \text{ min}} \times 15 \text{ gtt/ml}$$

◆ Divide the fraction and solve for X.

$$X = 1.39 \text{ ml/min} \times 15 \text{ gtt/ml}$$

$$X = 20.8 \text{ gtt/min}$$

The drip rate is 20.8 gtt/min, which can be rounded to 21 gtt/min.

A doctor's order calls for 1,000 ml of dextrose 5% in 0.45% sodium chloride I.V. over 10 hours. The solution will be infused through a Cutter administration set (drip factor is 20 gtt/ml). What is the flow rate (the amount infused in 1 hour) and the drip rate?

◆ To calculate the flow rate, set up the proportion and solve for X.

$$\frac{1,000 \text{ ml}}{10 \text{ hr}} = \frac{X \text{ ml}}{1 \text{ hr}}$$

$$10 \text{ hr} \times X \text{ ml} = 1,000 \text{ ml} \times 1 \text{ hr}$$

$$X = \frac{1,000 \text{ ml}}{10}$$

$$X = 100 \text{ ml}$$

The flow rate is 100 ml/hr.

◆ To find the drip rate, multiply the flow rate by the drip factor for the administration set, first converting 1 hour to 60 minutes.

$$X = \frac{100 \text{ ml}}{60 \text{ min}} \times \frac{20 \text{ gtt}}{1 \text{ ml}}$$

$$X = \frac{2,000 \text{ gtt}}{60 \text{ min}}$$

$$X = 33.3 \text{ gtt/min}$$

The flow rate is 33.3 gtt/min, which can be rounded to 33 gtt/min.

Rates for blood and blood products

The nurse can also use the formula method for calculations related to administration of blood and blood products.

The transfusion of blood and blood products requires special administration sets that contain filters to remove agglutinated cells. The drip factor for blood administration sets is usually 10 to 15 gtt/ml, and an 18G or larger needle is used for the I.V. insertion. These factors help prevent cell damage and ensure an adequate flow rate.

Most facilities have specific protocols for transfusing blood and blood products. For example, a unit of whole blood (about 500 ml) or packed red blood cells (about 250 ml) should infuse for no more than 4 hours because significant deterioration and bacterial contamination of the blood may occur after this time. Many facilities suggest that such a transfusion should be completed in about 2 hours. Note, however, that this rate may be too fast for pediatric and geriatric patients.

In addition, the nurse must take special precautions when transfusing blood products, such as platelets, cryoprecipitate, and granulocytes. Consult the facility's procedure manual to determine the type of tubing to use and the suggested rate and duration of the transfusion.

Patient situations

The doctor's order states Transfuse 1 unit packed red blood cells stat. *The patient is a young adult with no known cardiac impairment. The transfusion set has a drip factor of 15 gtt/ml. What is the transfusion rate (flow rate)? What is the drip rate?*

◆ To calculate the transfusion rate, set up the following proportion. For this calculation, assume that the facility requires the transfusion to be administered over 2 hours.

$$\frac{250 \text{ ml}}{2 \text{ hr}} = \frac{X \text{ ml}}{1 \text{ hr}}$$

$$X = 125 \text{ ml/hr}$$

◆ To calculate the drip rate, multiply the transfusion rate (flow rate) by the drip factor.

$$X = \frac{125 \text{ ml}}{60 \text{ min}} \times 15 \text{ gtt/ml}$$

$$X = \frac{1,875 \text{ gtt}}{60 \text{ min}}$$

$$X = 31.25, \text{ or } 31 \text{ gtt/min}$$

Note: Do not add blood or blood products to an I.V. line that contains a dextrose or calcium solution. A dextrose solution can cause cell hemolysis; a calcium solution, such as lactated Ringer's, can cause clotting. Normal saline solution is compatible with blood and blood products.

Using the formula method

Perform the following I.V. calculations, using the formula method. To check your answers, see page 198.

1. A patient needs to receive 500 ml of I.V. fluid over 6 hours. The I.V. drip factor is 10 gtt/ml. What is the drip rate?

2. The doctor prescribes 1,000 ml of I.V. fluid to be delivered over 24 hours. The nurse plans to use microdrip tubing. What is the drip rate?

3. The nurse prepares 250 ml of an I.V. solution, which will be delivered over 1 hour through an administration set with a drip factor of 15 gtt/ml. What is the drip rate?

4. A patient must receive 1,000 ml of I.V. fluid over 8 hours. The administration set's drip factor is 20 gtt/ml. What is the drip rate?

5. An order states *Give 2,000 ml of D$_5$NS I.V. over 8 hours.* The I.V. drip factor is 15 gtt/ml. What is the drip rate?

6. The doctor prescribes 1 unit of packed RBCs to be administered over 3 hours. The unit contains 250 ml, and the administration set's drip factor is 10 gtt/ml. What is the drip rate?

Using the division factor method

Instead of following all the steps required by the formula method, the nurse can use a quicker method to determine I.V. drip rates. This method is called the division factor (or short cut) method.

Drip rates

The division factor method takes advantage of the fact that all drip factors can be evenly divided into 60 to simplify the computation. For example, with a microdrip set (drip factor is 60 gtt/ml), the drip rate will equal the hourly flow rate. If the flow rate were 125 ml/60 minutes, the equation would be:

$$\text{Drip rate} = \frac{125 \text{ ml}}{60 \text{ min}} \times \frac{60 \text{ gtt}}{1 \text{ ml}}$$

$$\text{Drip rate} = 125 \text{ gtt/min}$$

In this example, the number of drops per minute (125) is the same as the number of milliliters of fluid per hour. Rather than spend time calculating the equation, the nurse can use the number assigned to the flow rate as the drip rate when using a microdrip set.

For I.V. administration sets that deliver 10 gtt/ml, divide the flow rate by 6 (which is known as the division factor) to find the drip rate. For sets that deliver 15 gtt/ml, divide the flow rate by 4 to find the drip rate. For sets that deliver 20 gtt/ml, divide the flow rate by 3 to find the drip rate. For example, if the ordered flow rate were 125 ml/hour with the solution infused through a Baxter administration set (drip factor of 10 gtt/ml), the equation would be:

$$\frac{125 \text{ ml}}{6} = 20.8 \text{ gtt/min}$$

In this example, the drip rate is 20.8 gtt/min, which can be rounded to 21 gtt/min. The drip rate obtained is the same whether this quick method or a longer one is used.

Patient situations

A doctor's order calls for 1,000 ml of D_5W to be infused over 12 hours. Determine the drip rate for an administration set that delivers 15 gtt/ml.

◆ To use the division factor method, begin by determining the flow rate. Divide the number of milliliters to be delivered by the number of hours.

$$X = \frac{1,000 \text{ ml}}{12 \text{ hr}}$$

$$X = 83.3 \text{ ml/hr}$$

◆ To find the drip rate, divide the flow rate by 4 (because the drip factor of the administration set is 15).

$$X = \frac{83.3}{4}$$

$$X = 20.8$$

The flow rate is 20.8 gtt/min, which can be rounded to 21 gtt/min.

A doctor's order states Infuse dextrose 5% in 0.33NS at 150 ml/hr. *The solution will be infused through a McGaw administration set (drip factor is 15 gtt/ml). What is the drip rate for 1 minute? What is the drip rate for 15 seconds?*

◆ Using the division factor method to calculate the drip rate for 1 minute, divide the flow rate by 4.

$$X = \frac{150 \text{ ml/hr}}{4}$$

$$X = 37.5, \text{ or } 38 \text{ gtt/min}$$

◆ To find the drip rate for 15 seconds, use the following equation.

$$X = \frac{38 \text{ gtt/min}}{4}$$

$$X = 9.5, \text{ or } 10 \text{ gtt/15 sec}$$

A doctor's order for a pediatric patient states **Infuse dextrose 5% in 0.25NS at 40 ml/hour. The solution will be infused through a microdrip administration tubing set (drip factor is 60 gtt/ml). What is the drip rate?**

♦ To find the drip rate, multiply the flow rate by the drip factor for the administration set.

$$X = \frac{40 \text{ ml}}{60 \text{ min}} \times \frac{60 \text{ gtt}}{1 \text{ ml}}$$

$$X = 40 \text{ gtt/min}$$

Because microdrip tubing will be used, the numerical value of the drip rate is equal to the numerical value of the flow rate. In this example, because the flow rate is 40, the drip rate also is 40.

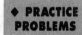

Using the division factor method

Answer the following questions about the division factor method. To check your answers, see page 198.

1. What is the division factor of an I.V. administration set with a drip factor of 15 gtt/ml?

2. If an I.V. administration set has a drip factor of 20 gtt/ml, what division factor should the nurse use?

3. The nurse has an administration set with a drip factor of 10 gtt/ml. What division factor should the nurse use?

4. Use the division factor method in these calculations.

   a) The nurse must administer I.V. fluid at 125 ml/hr. The drip factor is 15 gtt/ml. What is the drip rate?

   b) The doctor prescribes an I.V. to run at 150 ml/hr. The drip factor is 10 gtt/ml. What is the drip rate?

   c) The nurse is using an administration set with a drip factor of 60 gtt/ml to administer fluid at 42 ml/hr. What is the drip rate?

Regulating the infusion

After carefully calculating the drip rate using the formula or division factor method, the nurse must regulate the I.V. flow manually or electronically. If therapy calls for patient-controlled analgesia (PCA), the nurse sets up the infusion device and the patient regulates the dosage.

Manual regulation

The nurse manually regulates the I.V. drip rate by counting the number of drops that flow into the drip chamber. While counting the drops, the nurse adjusts the flow with the roller clamp until the fluid is infusing at the appropriate number of drops per minute.

Rather than counting for a full minute, however, the nurse may calculate the drip rate for 15 seconds and then count the drops in the chamber for 15 seconds. For example, if the prescribed drip rate is 31 gtt/min, the nurse divides 31 by 4 (because 15 seconds is ¼ of a minute) to get 8. Then the nurse adjusts the roller clamp until the drip chamber shows 8 drops in 15 seconds.

Electronic regulation

Electronic infusion devices, such as infusion controllers and infusion pumps, facilitate I.V. administration. (See *Electronic volumetric controller and electronic infusion pump* for photographs.) Infusion controllers regulate the rate of gravity-fed infusions by electronically counting or measuring drops or by determining the rate based on volume. Infusion pumps administer fluid under positive pressure and may be calibrated by drip rate or volume. Some new devices have variable pressure limits that prevent them from pumping fluids into infiltrated sites.

Electronic volumetric controller and electronic infusion pump

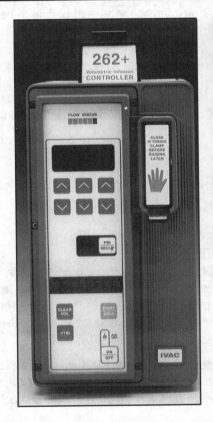 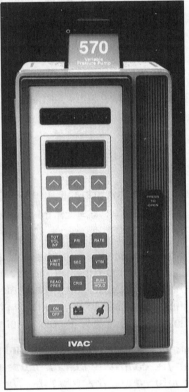

These devices permit the nurse to control the infusion rate by setting the volume or drip rate, shorten the time needed to calibrate an infusion rate, require less maintenance, and provide greater accuracy than the standard methods that drip fluid by gravity. Additionally, some devices keep track of the amount of fluid that has been infused, which helps the nurse maintain accurate intake and output records. Many devices include alarms that signal when the fluid container is empty or when a mechanical problem occurs.

The nurse sets the infusion device to deliver a constant amount of solution per minute or hour. Because each infusion device has its own operating instructions, follow the manufacturer's guidelines to ensure adequate functioning of the pump.

When working with a controller or pump, program it based on calculation of the infusion rate. An electronic infusion device does not eliminate the need for careful calculations and attention to infusion rates over time.

To determine the pump settings, consider the amount of fluid to be given and the time over which it must be infused. With most devices, the nurse must program the amount of fluid to be infused and the hourly flow rate. With others, the nurse must program the flow rate per minute or the drip rate.

Patient situations

A patient needs to receive 1,000 ml of fluid over 8 hours. How should the nurse set up the infusion pump?

♦ First, enter 1,000 ml into the infusion pump's program as the amount of fluid to be infused.

♦ Next, calculate the hourly flow rate.

$$X = \frac{1,000 \text{ ml}}{8 \text{ hr}}$$

$$X = 125 \text{ ml/hr}$$

♦ If using a device that requires calculation of the flow rate per minute, use the following equation.

$$X = \frac{125 \text{ ml}}{60 \text{ min}}$$

$$X = 2.1 \text{ ml/min}$$

♦ Finally, to calculate the drip rate, use the following equation.

$$X = 2.1 \text{ ml/min} \times 15 \text{ gtt/ml (drip factor)}$$

$$X = 31.5, \text{ or } 32 \text{ gtt/min}$$

Hint: Set the total volume to be infused at slightly less than the amount ordered. For example, if 1 L of fluid is ordered and hung, set the infusion device to 950 ml. Then, when the preset volume is reached (in this case, 950 ml) and the pump's alarm indicates that the next bottle should be hung, extra time to do so will be provided. Reset the infusion pump for the remaining amount of fluid (50 ml) and, while that is infusing, prepare the next I.V. bottle.

The doctor's order states Infuse 1,000 ml dextrose 5% in 0.33NS over 8 hours. The patient has an I.V. controller that the nurse must set with information about the volume of fluid to be infused and the drip rate. The drip factor is 10 gtt/ml. How should the nurse proceed?

♦ First, determine the hourly flow rate using this equation:

$$X = \frac{1,000 \text{ ml}}{8 \text{ hr}}$$

$$X = 125 \text{ ml/hr}$$

♦ Next, determine the flow rate per minute using this equation.

$$X = \frac{125 \text{ ml}}{60 \text{ min}}$$

$$X = 2.08 \text{ ml/min}$$

♦ Finally, calculate the drip rate by multiplying the flow rate by the drip factor.

$$X = 2.08, \text{ or } 2.1 \text{ ml/min} \times 10 \text{ gtt/ml}$$

$$X = 20.8, \text{ or } 21 \text{ gtt/min}$$

Set the volume of fluid to be infused at 1,000 ml and the drip rate at 21 gtt/minute.

A geriatric patient is to receive 250 ml of packed RBCs over 4 hours. This will be administered via an I.V. pump that requires the nurse to set the flow rate. How should the nurse set the pump?

♦ To calculate the flow rate, set up the following equation.

$$\frac{250 \text{ ml}}{4 \text{ hr}} = \frac{X \text{ ml}}{1 \text{ hr}}$$

$$X = 62.5, \text{ or } 63 \text{ ml/hr}$$

The flow rate on the pump should be set at 63 ml/hour.

PCA

PCA devices are specially designed I.V. infusion pumps that allow patients to self-administer analgesic medication. (See *PCA infusion pump* for an example.) The computerized pump, which is attached to the patient's I.V. line, is programmed by the nurse (or, in some situations, by the patient or caregiver) to deliver a precise dose of pain medication, usually morphine, when the patient pushes the control button. PCA pumps can also be programmed to deliver a basal dose of the medication in addition to the patient-controlled dose.

PCA infusion pump

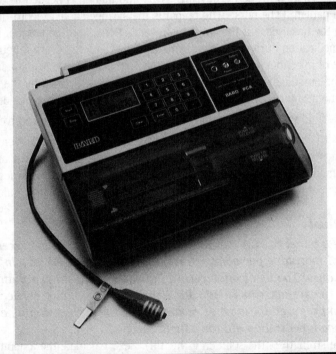

PCA devices provide consistent blood concentrations of pain medication and are considered superior to the traditional pain-relief approach, in which the nurse administers analgesic medication every few hours, usually by the intramuscular route. The traditional approach produces fluctuating blood levels of analgesic medication, resulting in periods of heavy sedation alternating with periods of increasing pain. An added benefit of PCA devices is that patients tend to take less medication than they would with the more traditional approach. PCA also is considered superior to continuous I.V. infusion of analgesic medication because the patient gains a measure of pain control.

Several safety features are built into PCA devices. For example, the medication dose and administration frequency are programmed into the machine. If the patient requests medication too frequently, the machine ignores the requests, thus preventing overdose. Furthermore, some machines record both filled and unfilled requests for medication; the PCA's log shows the number of attempts and the number of times the patient actually received the medication. Thus, the nurse will know if the patient is continually requesting medication and can evaluate the need for it.

PCA devices require use of an access code or key before drug dose and frequency information can be entered into the system. This prevents accidental resetting or tampering with the device by unauthorized persons. In addition, some machines record unauthorized entries.

When caring for a patient receiving PCA, follow these guidelines:

• Draw up the correct amount and concentration of medication, and insert it into the PCA device.

• Program the device according to the manufacturer's directions (an average setting is 1 mg of morphine every 6 minutes or longer).

• Read and interpret the PCA log, and record the information on the patient's medication record.

When interpreting the PCA log, note the strength (the number of milligrams per milliliter) of the medication solution in the PCA syringe. This information is needed to calculate the dose received by the patient. (The nurse who prepares the syringe should record the solution's strength.) Note the basal dose if the patient is receiving one, and the number of times the patient received medication during the time being assessed (usually every 4 hours). By multiplying the number of injections received by the volume of each injection (and adding the basal dose, if any), the nurse can determine the amount of solution received by the patient. Then multiply this amount by the strength of the solution, as shown in this equation:

$$\text{fluid volume} \times \text{solution strength} = \text{total medication received}$$

Record the result (the milligrams of drug received) in the patient's medication record.

Most facilities require the nurse who prepares the syringe to record the amount of fluid and the amount of medication in the syringe. Each nurse who checks the PCA log also records this information. The data enable nurses to double-check the accuracy of their calculations.

Patient situations

When reading a patient's PCA log, the nurse notes that the patient received a basal dose of 1 ml of morphine per hour and requested and received four injections of 2 ml each, over 4 hours. The medication record indicates that 1 ml of solution contains 1 mg of morphine. The syringe was filled with 30 ml of fluid 4 hours earlier; 18 ml remain. The nurse who prepared the syringe recorded that the syringe contained 30 mg of morphine. How much medication did the patient receive?

◆ First, note the strength of the solution (1 mg/ml). Next, calculate the amount of fluid received via the basal rate:

$$4 \text{ hr} \times 1 \text{ ml/hr} = 4 \text{ ml}$$

◆ Next, calculate the amount of fluid received on demand:

$$4 \text{ injections} \times 2 \text{ ml} = 8 \text{ ml}$$

◆ Then, calculate the total amount of fluid received by adding the basal and demand dosages:

$$4 \text{ ml (basal)} + 8 \text{ ml (demand)} = 12 \text{ ml}$$

◆ To determine the amount of morphine the patient received, use the equation:

$$12 \text{ ml} \times 1 \text{ mg/ml} = 12 \text{ mg}$$

To double-check, subtract the amount of fluid received (12 ml) from the amount in the syringe at the last log check (30 ml). The result should equal the amount remaining in the device (18 ml). Or double-check the calculations based on the actual medication dosage. The syringe originally contained 30 mg of morphine with a strength of 1 mg/ml. Since the patient received 12 mg, then 18 mg (18 ml) should remain.

A patient is receiving morphine via a PCA device. The medication record indicates that 1 ml of solution contains 1 mg of morphine. When reading the PCA, the nurse notes that the device is set to deliver a basal rate of 2 ml/hour. In addition to this, the patient requested and received two injections of 1 ml each, over 4 hours. The syringe contained 20 ml of fluid at the beginning of the shift. How much medication did the patient receive over the 4-hour period? How much fluid should remain in the syringe?

◆ First, calculate the amount of medication received via the basal rate.

$$X = 4 \text{ hr} \times 2 \text{ mg/hr}$$
$$X = 8 \text{ mg}$$

◆ Next, calculate the amount of medication received on demand.

$$X = 2 \text{ requests} \times 1 \text{ mg/request}$$
$$X = 2 \text{ mg}$$

◆ Add the basal and demand medication dosages to determine the total amount of medication received.

$$X = 8 \text{ mg (basal)} + 2 \text{ mg (demand)}$$
$$X = 10 \text{ mg}$$

◆ Because the strength of the solution is 1 mg/ml, the patient received 10 ml of fluid. Subtract to determine the amount of fluid remaining in the syringe.

$$X = 20 \text{ ml} - 10 \text{ ml}$$

10 ml of fluid should remain in the syringe. If not, check the calculations.

◆ **PRACTICE PROBLEMS**	## Regulating the infusion

Answer the following questions about regulating I.V. infusions. To check your answers, see page 199.

1. The nurse needs to administer an I.V. infusion at 63 gtt/min. When manually regulating the infusion, how many drops should the nurse count in 15 seconds?

2. An I.V. infusion is to run at 25 gtt/min. When manually regulating the infusion, how many drops should the nurse see in 15 seconds?

3. How many drops of I.V. fluid should the nurse count in 15 seconds, if the drip rate is 42 gtt/min?

4. For an I.V. infusion, the nurse calculates the drip rate to be 28 gtt/min. What should the 15-second rate be?

5. The doctor prescribes I.V. fluid to run at 10 gtt/min. What should the 15-second rate be?

6. The doctor prescribes 1,000 ml of dextrose 5% in 0.9% sodium chloride to run over 10 hours, using an I.V. controller. The nurse must set the volume to be infused and the drip rate in drops/minute. The drip factor is 20 gtt/ml. What is the volume to be infused and the drip rate?

7. A patient needs to receive 3 L of dextrose 5% in ½ NS over 24 hours. The fluid is to be infused via an I.V. pump that requires the nurse to set the hourly rate and volume. How should the nurse set the pump?

8. The doctor's order states, *Infuse 500 ml of NS over 2 hours.* What volume should the nurse set on the pump? What hourly rate should the nurse set?

9. A patient must receive 1,000 ml of D_5W at 83 ml/hr. The fluid will be administered via an I.V. controller that requires the nurse to set the drip rate. The drip factor is 15 gtt/ml. What is the drip rate?

10. A patient has been receiving morphine via a PCA device, in a strength of 1 mg/ml. The PCA log shows that the patient received 4 doses of 1 ml each over 4 hours in addition to a basal dose of 2 mg/hr. How many milligrams of morphine did the patient receive in those 4 hours?

Adjusting the infusion rate

Although the nurse carefully calculates the I.V. drip rate and adjusts the flow according to the 15-second drop count, the I.V. rate may change for a number of reasons. For example, patient position changes, kinked I.V. tubing, or infiltration at the I.V. site can cause the infusion to run ahead of or behind schedule. When this occurs, the nurse must recalculate the drip rate, using the remaining time and volume.

Patient situation

A patient was supposed to receive 1,000 ml of NS over 8 hours. The nurse used an administration set with a drip factor of 10 gtt/ml, and set the drip rate at 21 gtt/min. After 4 hours, the nurse finds that only 250 ml have been infused, instead of the 500 ml that should have been infused. Now the nurse must recalculate the drip rate for the remaining solution.

♦ First, use the remaining time (4 hours) and volume (750 ml) to determine the flow rate.

$$\frac{750 \text{ ml}}{4 \text{ hr}} = 187.5 \text{ or } 188 \text{ ml/hr}$$

The new flow rate is 188 ml/hr.

♦ Next, calculate the drip rate based on the flow rate and drip factor, which is 10 gtt/ml in this case.

To calculate the flow rate per minute, use the following equation.

$$X = \frac{188 \text{ ml}}{60 \text{ min}}$$

$$X = 3.1 \text{ ml/min}$$

To calculate the drip rate, use the following equation.

$$X = 3.1 \text{ ml/min} \times 10 \text{ gtt/ml}$$
$$X = 31 \text{ gtt/min}$$

So the nurse should increase the drip rate to 31 gtt/min to administer the solution on time. *Note:* If I.V. fluid has been infused too quickly, the nurse should assess the patient for signs of fluid overload, such as crackles and increased blood pressure. If fluid has been infused too slowly, the nurse should assess the patient to determine if he can tolerate an increased rate. To do this, the nurse assesses his cardiac and respiratory status and checks for a history of renal insufficiency, pulmonary edema, or any other condition that increases the risk of fluid overload.

Fluid challenge

Besides adjusting the rate to keep an infusion on schedule, the nurse may need to alter the infusion rate in response to the doctor's order. The doctor may wish to evaluate a patient's response to an increased intake of fluids, sometimes referred to as a "fluid challenge." This can be accomplished most quickly by increasing the flow rate of the I.V. infusion for a specified time and then reducing it to a maintenance rate. (*Note:* Use caution when greatly increasing the infusion rate in pediatric and geriatric patients.)

Patient situation

A patient is to receive a fluid challenge of 500 ml of normal saline over 2 hours. The administration set has a drip factor of 15 gtt/ml. What should the flow rate and drip rate be?

◆ To calculate the flow rate, set up the proportion.

$$\frac{500 \text{ ml}}{2 \text{ hr}} = \frac{X \text{ ml}}{1 \text{ hr}}$$
$$2X = 500$$
$$X = 250 \text{ ml/hr}$$

◆ To calculate the drip rate, multiply the flow rate by the drip factor of the administration set.

$$X = \frac{250 \text{ ml}}{60 \text{ min}} \times \frac{15 \text{ gtt}}{1 \text{ ml}}$$

$$X = \frac{3,750 \text{ gtt}}{60 \text{ min}}$$

$$X = 62.5, \text{ or } 63 \text{ gtt/min}$$

Thus, the solution should infuse at 63 gtt/min in order to deliver the fluid challenge.

◆ PRACTICE PROBLEMS

Adjusting the infusion rate

Answer the following questions about adjusting infusion rates. To check your answers, see page 199.

1. A patient is supposed to receive 1,000 ml of D_5NS over 12 hours. The administration set has a drip factor of 15 gtt/ml. What is the drip rate?

After 6 hours, the nurse notices that 650 ml of fluid have been infused. After the nurse recalculates the rate for the remaining fluid, what should the drip rate be?

2. The doctor prescribes normal saline (0.9% NaCl) I.V. at 500 ml/hr for 1 hour, followed by a maintenance dosage of 150 ml/hr. The drip factor is 10 gtt/ml. What is the drip rate during the first hour? What is the drip rate for the maintenance dosage?

3. A patient needs to receive 1,000 ml of D_5W I.V. over 6 hours. The drip factor is 20 gtt/ml. What is the drip rate? After 4 hours, the nurse discovers that only 500 ml of fluid have been infused. After recalculation, what is the drip rate?

4. The doctor orders a fluid challenge of 250 ml of normal saline (0.9% NaCl) I.V. over 1 hour, followed by a maintenance infusion of 100 ml/hr. The drip factor is 15 gtt/ml. What is the drip rate during the fluid challenge? What is the drip rate of the maintenance infusion?

5. A patient is supposed to receive 1,000 ml of D5 0.9 NS I.V. over 8 hours. The nurse sets up the infusion with an administration set that has a drip factor of 15 gtt/ml. After 6 hours, 400 ml of fluid remain in the I.V. bag. After recalculation, what drip rate should the nurse use to get the infusion back on schedule?

Review problems

Answer the following questions related to I.V. flow rates. To check your answers, see page 199.

1. The drip rate refers to the number of drops per _____ .

2. The drip factor for a microdrip administration set is _____ .

3. The doctor orders 2,000 ml of D_5LR I.V. over the first 24 hours postoperatively. The administration set has a drip factor of 15 gtt/ml. How many drops per minute should be delivered?

4. A patient is to receive 1 L of I.V. lactated Ringer's solution over 10 hours. A set with a drip factor of 10 gtt/ml is to be used. What should the drip rate be?

5. A patient must receive 1,000 ml of D_5NS over 4 hours. From a set with a drip factor of 20 gtt/ml, how many drops per minute should the patient receive?

6. If a patient's I.V. infusion is dripping at 31 gtt/min and the set has a drip factor of 15 gtt/ml, how many milliliters will the patient receive during an 8-hour shift?

7. The doctor orders I.V. dextrose 5% in ⅓NS at 80 ml/hr. A set with a drip factor of 20 gtt/ml is to be used. What should the drip rate be?

8. If a child is to receive 30 ml/hr of dextrose 5% in ¼ NS I.V. through a minidrip delivery set, what should the drip rate be?

9. If a patient needs to receive 500 ml of dextrose 5% in ½ NS I.V. over 24 hours through a microdrip set, what will the drip rate be?

10. If a patient must receive maintenance I.V. dosing at 15 gtt/min through a microdrip set, how many milliliters will the patient receive in 8 hours?

11. The doctor's order reads *Administer 1,000 ml dextrose 5% in 0.45NS c̄ 40 mEq of KCl over 6 hours.* The available administration set has a drip factor of 15 gtt/ml. What should the drip rate be?

12. If a patient is to receive 100 ml/hour I.V. and the drip factor is 15 gtt/ml, how many drops per minute should the nurse set the administration set to deliver?

13. The nurse manually regulates the I.V. drip rate by counting the number of drops that flow into the _____ .

14. An I.V. infusion is to run at 24 gtt/min. When manually regulating the infusion, how many drops should the nurse see in 15 seconds?

15. A patient needs to receive 1 L of dextrose 5% in ½ NS over 4 hours. The fluid is to be infused via an I.V. pump that requires the nurse to set the hourly rate. How should the nurse set the pump?

16. The doctor orders a 200 ml I.V. fluid challenge over 30 minutes, followed by a regular infusion rate of 100 ml/hour. If the drip factor is 10 gtt/ml, what will the drip rate be for the fluid challenge? The regular I.V. infusion?

17. A patient needs to receive 400 ml normal saline I.V. over 1 hour, followed by regular infusion rate of 50 ml/hr. The set has a drip factor of 15 gtt/ml. What would the drip rate be for the first hour? What would the drip rate be after the first hour?

18. The doctor orders a 300 ml I.V. fluid challenge over 30 minutes, followed by a regular infusion rate of 1 L over 10 hours. If the drip factor is 10 gtt/ml, what will the drip rate be for the fluid challenge? What will the drip rate be for the infusion?

19. A patient is to receive 200 ml normal saline I.V. over 15 minutes, followed by normal saline I.V. at 100 ml/hr. The set has a drip factor of 10 gtt/ml. For the first 15 minutes, what would the drip rate be? After the first 15 minutes, what would the drip rate be?

20. The doctor prescribes a 250 ml I.V. fluid challenge over 30 minutes, followed by a regular infusion rate of 75 ml/hour. If the drip factor is 10 gtt/ml, what will the drip rate be for the fluid challenge? For the regular infusion?

21. A patient is to receive 275 ml of packed RBCs over 2 hours. The set has a drip factor of 10 gtt/ml. What should the drip rate of the transfusion be?

22. The doctor orders 1 unit of packed RBCs to infuse over 4 hours. The unit contains 250 ml, and the set has a drip factor of 15 gtt/ml. What should the drip rate be?

23. A patient must receive 100 ml of platelets over 15 minutes. The set has a drip factor of 15 gtt/ml. What should the drip rate of the transfusion be?

24. After 4 hours, the nurse checks a patient's PCA log and notes that the patient requested and received three doses of 1 ml each. The nurse notes that each milliliter contains 1 mg of morphine. How many milligrams of morphine did the patient receive over the 4 hours?

25. At the beginning of the shift, the nurse notes that 30 ml of morphine remain in a patient's PCA device. The PCA record shows that the morphine dosage strength is 2 mg/ml. After 2 hours, the nurse checks the PCA log and notes that the patient made six attempts and received five doses of 1 ml each. How many milligrams of morphine did the patient receive in 2 hours?

26. At the beginning of the shift, the nurse notes that 50 ml of morphine remain in a patient's PCA device. The PCA record shows that the morphine dosage strength is 2 mg/ml, and that the device is set to administer a basal dose of 2 mg/hr. After 4 hours, the nurse checks the PCA log and notes that the patient made 12 attempts and received 10 doses of 1 ml each on demand. How many milligrams of morphine did the patient receive in 4 hours?

27. A patient needs to receive 3 L of fluid over 24 hours via I.V. pump. The pump requires the nurse to set the hourly rate and the volume of fluid to be infused. The nurse is to hang the first 1-L bag of solution at 9 A.M. How should the nurse proceed?

28. The doctor's order states: *1 L D_5W – infuse at 125 ml/hr.* This fluid will be administered via an I.V. controller that requires the nurse to set the drip rate. (The administration set has a drip factor of 15 gtt/ml.) How should the nurse proceed?

29. A patient is supposed to receive 500 ml of D5 ¼ normal saline I.V. over 6 hours. The drip factor is 20 gtt/ml. After 2 hours, the nurse finds that 250 ml have been infused. After re-calculation, what is the drip rate?

30. The doctor orders 1 L of normal saline to run over 8 hours. The drip factor is 20 gtt/ml. After 3 hours, the nurse finds 300 ml remain to be infused. What is the drip rate after recalculation?

31. A patient must receive 1 L of D_5W over 10 hours. The drip factor is 15 gtt/ml. After 4 hours, 400 ml remain in the bag. To get the infusion back on schedule, how should the nurse set the drip rate?

Answers to practice problems

◆ Identifying I.V. drip factors
1. drip rate
2. drip factor
3. a) 15 gtt/ml
   b) 20 gtt/ml
   c) 10 gtt/ml
   d) 12 gtt/min

◆ Using the formula method
1. 13.8 or 14 gtt/min
2. 41.7 or 42 gtt/min
3. 62.5 or 63 gtt/min
4. 41.7 or 42 gtt/min
5. 62.5 or 63 gtt/min
6. 13.8 or 14 gtt/min

◆ Using the division factor method
1. 4
2. 3
3. 6
4. a) 31.25 or 31 gtt/min
   b) 25 gtt/min
   c) 42 gtt/min

◆ *Regulating the infusion*

1. 15.75 or 16 gtt
2. 6.25 or 6 gtt
3. 10.5 or 10 gtt
4. 7 gtt
5. 2.5 or 3 gtt
6. 1,000 ml; 33.3 or 33 gtt/min
7. 125 ml/hr; 1,000 ml
8. 500 ml; 250 ml/hr
9. 20.75 or 21 gtt/min
10. 12 mg

◆ *Adjusting the infusion rate*

1. 20.8 or 21 gtt/min; 14.6 or 15 gtt/min
2. 83.3 or 83 gtt/min; 25 gtt/min
3. 55.6 or 56 gtt/min; 83.3 or 83 gtt/min
4. 62.5 or 63 gtt/min; 25 gtt/min
5. 50 gtt/min

Answers to review problems

1. minute
2. 60 gtt/ml
3. 20.8 or 21 gtt/min
4. 16.6 or 17 gtt/min
5. 83.3 or 83 gtt/min
6. 993.6 ml, rounded to 1,000 ml
7. 26.6 or 27 gtt/min
8. 30 gtt/min
9. 20.8 or 21 gtt/min
10. 120 ml
11. 41.6 or 42 gtt/min
12. 25 gtt/min
13. drip chamber
14. 6 gtt
15. 250 ml/hr
16. For the fluid challenge, 66.6 or 67 gtt/min; for the regular infusion, 16.6 or 17 gtt/min

17. For the first hour, 100 gtt/min; after the first hour, 12.5 or 13 gtt/min

18. For the fluid challenge, 100 gtt/min; for the regular infusion, 16.6 or 17 gtt/min

19. For the first 15 minutes, 133.3 or 133 gtt/min; after the first 15 minutes, 16.6 or 17 gtt/min

20. For the fluid challenge, 83.3 or 83 gtt/min; for the regular infusion, 12.5 or 13 gtt/min

21. 22.9 or 23 gtt/min

22. 15.6 or 16 gtt/min

23. 99.9 or 100 gtt/min

24. 3 mg

25. 10 mg

26. 28 mg

27. Set the flow rate at 125 ml/hr and the volume at 1,000 ml. The infusion should begin at 9 A.M. (The first liter will be completed at 5 P.M.)

28. Set the drip rate at 31.2 or 31 gtt/min.

29. 20.8 or 21 gtt/min

30. 20 gtt/min

31. 16.6 or 17 gtt/min

Chapter

18

I.V. Infusion Time Calculations

In addition to calculating the flow rate of an intravenous (I.V.) solution, the nurse must be able to compute the *infusion time* (time required for a certain volume of I.V. fluid to be infused). Determining the infusion time helps the nurse keep the infusion on schedule and ensure timely preparation of the next I.V. solution. It also allows the nurse to perform—as scheduled—laboratory tests associated with the infusion, such as those commonly ordered for patients receiving total parenteral nutrition. (For details, see *Understanding TPN*.)

To help you master these skills, Chapter 18 demonstrates how to calculate infusion times and use this information to time-tape the I.V. fluid container.

Understanding TPN

A patient receives total parenteral nutrition (TPN) when nutrient needs cannot be met enterally because of elevated requirements or impaired digestion or absorption in the GI tract. TPN—also called central parenteral nutrition (CPN) or intravenous hyperalimentation (IVH or HAL)—can be administered centrally via the superior vena cava, inferior vena cava, or right atrium, or peripherally via the veins of the arms, legs, or scalp. Most facilities have a written protocol regarding insertion sites and recommended solutions.

TPN is available as commercially prepared products or individually formulated solutions from the pharmacy. The solutions are prepared under sterile and carefully monitored conditions to guard against patient infection. Nurses rarely are responsible for preparing these solutions on the patient unit.

TPN solutions contain a 10% or greater dextrose concentration. Amino acids are provided to maintain or restore nitrogen balance, and vitamins, electrolytes, and trace minerals are added to meet individual needs. Lipids also are provided but are given separately to prevent their destruction by the other nutrients. (*Note:* Because additives increase a solution's total volume, they affect intake measurements. For example, when assessing the amount of fluid remain-

(continued)

Understanding TPN (continued)

ing in the patient's TPN bottle, the nurse may find 20 to 50 ml more than expected. In that case, determine whether the volume of additives explains the discrepancy.)

Initially, TPN is infused at a slow rate, which is gradually increased to a maintenance level. Similarly, the rate is gradually decreased before discontinuing TPN. Most TPN solutions are administered via infusion pump.

Patient situation

A patient with cancer of the GI tract is receiving TPN. The doctor's order states 500 ml 8.5% Aminosyn + 500 ml 20% dextrose I.V. with 1 ampule trace elements + 1 ampule multivitamins + 1 ampule MgSO₄ to infuse over 6 hours. The solution was hung at 7:00 A.M. How many milliliters remain at 11:00 A.M.?

♦ First, calculate the hourly flow rate.

$$X = \frac{1,000 \text{ ml}}{6 \text{ hr}}$$

$$X = 166.67, \text{ or } 167 \text{ ml/hr}$$

♦ Next, calculate the amount of solution that should have been administered by 11:00 A.M. Because the solution has been infusing for 4 hours at 167 ml/hour, the equation would be:

$$X = 4 \text{ hr} \times 167 \text{ ml/hr}$$

$$X = 668, \text{ or } 670 \text{ ml}$$

♦ Next, calculate the amount of fluid remaining by subtracting the amount of fluid infused from the amount of solution hung.

$$\begin{array}{r} 1,000 \text{ ml} \\ - \quad 670 \text{ ml} \\ \hline 330 \text{ ml} \end{array}$$

Thus, 330 ml should remain in the bottle at 11:00 A.M. The nurse may note, however, that 350 ml remain. The ampules of additives (trace elements, multivitamins, and MgSO₄) may explain the discrepancy.

Using the infusion-time formula

To calculate the infusion time, the nurse must know the flow rate (ml/hr) and the volume to be infused. (For details, see Chapter 17, I.V. Flow Rate Calculations.)

Infusion time = volume to be infused (in ml) ÷ flow rate (ml/hr)

Patient situations

A patient needs to receive 1 L of NS I.V. at 40 ml/hr. What is the infusion time?

♦ First, set up the formula with the information for this patient. (Remember to convert the volume into milliliters, if needed.)

Infusion time = 1,000 ml ÷ 40 ml/hr

◆ Then perform the arithmetic, canceling out the milliliters in the numerator and denominator.

$$\text{Infusion time} = 1{,}000 \text{ ml} \times \frac{1 \text{ hr}}{40 \text{ ml}}$$

$$\text{Infusion time} = 25 \text{ hr}$$

The infusion time is 25 hours for this patient.

The doctor orders 500 ml of D_5W to run at 42 ml/hr. What is the infusion time?
◆ First, set up the formula with the appropriate information.

$$\text{Infusion time} = 500 \text{ ml} \div 42 \text{ ml/hr}$$

◆ Then perform the arithmetic, canceling out the milliliters in the numerator and denominator.

$$\text{Infusion time} = 500 \text{ ml} \times \frac{1 \text{ hr}}{42 \text{ ml}}$$

$$\text{Infusion time} = 11.9 \text{ hr}$$

◆ Finally, convert the decimal fraction (.9) to minutes. To do this, multiply by 60 because 60 minutes equal 1 hour.

$$.9 \times 60 = 54 \text{ min}$$

So the infusion time is 11 hours, 54 minutes.

A patient is to receive an I.V. of 1,000 ml D_5NS to run at 90 ml/hr. After 750 ml have been infused, the nurse must draw a blood sample from the patient and send it to the laboratory to determine electrolyte levels. The infusion begins at 9 A.M. When should the nurse draw the blood from the patient?
◆ For this patient, you need to know the infusion time of the first 750 ml of I.V. fluid. So set up the formula, using that information.

$$\text{Infusion time} = 750 \text{ ml} \div 90 \text{ ml/hr}$$

◆ Then perform the arithmetic, canceling out the milliliters in the numerator and denominator.

$$\text{Infusion time} = 750 \text{ ml} \times \frac{1 \text{ hr}}{90 \text{ ml}}$$

$$\text{Infusion time} = 8.3 \text{ hr}$$

◆ Finally, convert the decimal fraction (.3) to minutes by multiplying it times 60.

$$.3 \times 60 = 18 \text{ min}$$

The infusion time is 8 hours, 18 minutes. Because the infusion began at 9 A.M., the nurse should draw the blood sample 8 hours, 18 minutes later—at 5:18 P.M. (For more information on monitoring infusion rates, see *Time-taping an I.V. solution*, page 204.)

◆ PRACTICE PROBLEMS	**Using the infusion-time formula**

Answer the following questions about using the infusion-time formula. To check your answers, see pages 207 and 208.

1. At 9 A.M., the nurse starts an I.V. infusion, which is set to deliver 1 L at 125 ml/hr. What is the infusion time? When will the infusion be complete?

2. The doctor prescribes 1 L of normal saline I.V. to run at 200 ml/hr. What is the infusion time? If the I.V. is hung at 2 A.M., when will it be complete?

Time-taping an I.V. solution

To ensure that an I.V. solution is administered at the prescribed rate and to facilitate the recording of fluid intake, time-tape the bag. Some facilities require the nurse to do this and may provide labels for this purpose.

To time-tape an I.V. bag, place a piece of adhesive tape from the top to the bottom of the bag, next to the markings that indicate fluid level (see the illustration below, which shows a bag time-taped for a rate of 100 ml/hour). Next to the "0" marking, record the time that the bag was hung. Then, knowing the hourly rate, mark each hour on the tape next to the corresponding fluid marking. At the bottom of the tape, mark the time at which the solution will be completely infused. (Do not write directly on I.V. bags with felt-tip markers because the ink may seep into the I.V. fluid. Some manufacturers provide printed time tapes for use with their solutions.)

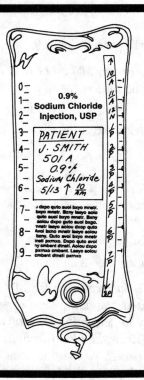

3. A patient needs to receive 250 ml of normal saline I.V. at 42 ml/hr. What is the infusion time?

4. A patient must receive 150 ml of D₅W to run at 25 ml/hr. What is the infusion time? If the infusion begins at 11 A.M., when will it be complete?

5. The doctor's order states, *Hang 1 L of D₅NS to run at 150 ml/hr. Draw blood for electrolyte levels after 500 ml have been infused.* The nurse starts the infusion at 11 A.M. When should the nurse draw the blood sample?

6. A patient receives parenteral nutrition when _____ needs cannot be met enterally.

7. A burn patient is receiving TPN. The doctor's order states *500 ml 8.5% Aminosyn, plus 500 ml 20% dextrose I.V., 1 ampule trace elements, 1 ampule multivitamins, and 1 ampule MgSO₄ to infuse over 8 hours.* The nurse hangs the solution at 8 A.M. How many milliliters should remain in the bag at 2 P.M.?

8. The doctor orders 1 L of D₅W I.V. to run at 125 ml/hr. Before handing the bag, the nurse writes 9 A.M. on the I.V. time-tape next to the "0" mark. What time should be written at the bottom of the time-tape, indicating when the infusion should be completed?

9. The nurse should not write infusion time information directly on I.V. bags with felt-tip markers because the ink may _____ _____ the I.V. fluid.

Adapting the infusion-time formula

If the only available information is the volume to be infused, drip factor, and drip rate, the nurse can still use the infusion-time formula to determine the infusion time. However, the nurse must first adapt it by converting the drip rate (gtt/min) to a flow rate (ml/hr).

Patient situation

The nurse must administer 1 L of D$_5$W I.V. at 31 gtt/min, using an administration set with a drip factor of 15 gtt/ml. What is the infusion time?

◆ First, convert the drip rate (gtt/min) to ml/min, using a proportion with ratios.

$$15 \text{ gtt} : 1 \text{ ml} :: 31 \text{ gtt} : X \text{ ml}$$
$$15 \times X = 1 \times 31$$
$$15X = 31$$
$$X = \frac{31}{15}$$
$$X = 2.06 \text{ ml/min, rounded to 2 ml/min}$$

◆ Next, convert 2 ml/min to the flow rate (ml/hr). To do this, simply multiply by 60 because 60 minutes equal 1 hour.

$$2 \text{ ml/min} \times 60 \text{ min} = 120 \text{ ml/hr}$$

◆ Then, calculate the infusion time, using the infusion-time formula.

$$\text{Infusion time} = 1,000 \text{ ml} \div 120 \text{ ml/hr}$$
$$\text{Infusion time} = 1,000 \text{ ml} \times \frac{1 \text{ hr}}{120 \text{ ml}}$$
$$\text{Infusion time} = 8.3 \text{ hr}$$

◆ Finally, convert the decimal fraction (.3) to minutes by multiplying it times 60.

$$.3 \times 60 = 18 \text{ min}$$

The infusion time is 8 hours, 18 minutes.

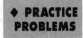

Adapting the infusion-time formula

Perform the following calculations, adapting the infusion-time formula as needed. To check your answers, see page 208.

1. The nurse must administer 1 L of NS at 50 gtt/min, using an administration set with a drip factor of 20 gtt/ml. What is the infusion time?

2. A patient must receive 1 L of D$_5$W ½NS I.V. at 21 gtt/min. The administration set has a drip factor of 15 gtt/ml. What is the infusion time?

3. The doctor's order states *500 ml of 20% Liposyn at 21 gtt/min.* The available administration set has a drip factor of 20 gtt/ml. What is the infusion time?

4. The nurse must administer 1 L of D$_5$NS at 25 gtt/min. The administration set has a drip factor of 10 gtt/ml. What is the infusion time?

5. The doctor orders 250 ml of NS at 62 gtt/min. The nurse uses an administration set with a drip factor of 15 gtt/ml. What is the infusion time?

Using the alternative formula method

Instead of adapting the infusion-time formula when only the volume to be infused, drip rate, and drip factor are known, the nurse may prefer to use this special formula.

$$\text{Infusion time} = \frac{\text{volume to be infused}}{(\text{drip rate/drip factor}) \times 60 \text{ min}}$$

Patient situation

A doctor prescribes 500 ml of NS I.V. at 32 gtt/min. The drip factor is 15 gtt/ml. What is the infusion time?

◆ First, set up the formula with the known information.

$$\text{Infusion time} = \frac{500 \text{ ml}}{(32 \text{ gtt/min/15 gtt/ml}) \times 60 \text{ min}}$$

◆ Then simplify the denominator and round it off, if necessary.

$$\text{Infusion time} = \frac{500 \text{ ml}}{2.13 \text{ ml/min} \times 60 \text{ min}}$$

$$\text{Infusion time} = \frac{500 \text{ ml}}{127.8 \text{ ml/hr}}$$

$$\text{Infusion time} = \frac{500 \text{ ml}}{128 \text{ ml/hr}}$$

◆ Divide the denominator into the numerator.

$$\text{Infusion time} = 3.9 \text{ hr}$$

◆ Finally, convert the decimal fraction (.9) into minutes by multiplying it times 60.

$$.9 \times 60 \text{ min} = 54 \text{ min}$$

The infusion time is 3 hours, 54 minutes.

◆ PRACTICE PROBLEMS

Using the alternative formula method

Perform the following calculations, using the alternate formula method. To check your answers, see page 208.

1. The doctor's order reads, *Infuse 100 ml D₅W IVPB at 67 gtt/min.* The administration set's drip factor is 20 gtt/ml. What is the infusion time? If the nurse starts the infusion at 9 A.M., when will it be complete?

2. The nurse must administer 1 L of D₅W I.V. at 24 gtt/min. The drip factor is 20 gtt/ml. What is the infusion time? If the nurse starts the infusion at 10 A.M., when will it be complete?

3. The doctor prescribes 500 ml of D₅RL (Dextrose 5% and Ringer's lactate) to run at 36 gtt/min. The drip factor is 10 gtt/ml. What is the infusion time?

4. A patient needs to receive 1 L of normal saline at 21 gtt/min. The nurse selects an administration set with a drip factor of 15 gtt/ml. What is the infusion time?

5. A patient is to receive 125 ml of cryoprecipitate, which is to be infused at 42 gtt/min through a set with a drip factor of 15 gtt/ml. What is the infusion time?

Review problems

Answer the following questions about infusion times. To check your answers, see page 208.

1. What term describes the total time required for a certain volume of I.V. fluid to be infused?

2. When enteral nutrition cannot meet a patient's nutritional needs, what is the doctor most likely to prescribe?

3. A patient must receive 6 units of platelets, which are contained in a 330-ml bag, at a rate of 150 ml/hr. What is the infusion time? If the nurse starts the transfusion at 5 P.M., when will it be complete?

4. At 2:00 A.M., a patient's I.V. therapy began and is scheduled to deliver 1 L of normal saline at 225 ml/hr. After 500 ml have been infused, the nurse must draw a blood sample for laboratory tests. When should the nurse draw the blood?

5. The patient is to receive 1 L of D5 ½ normal saline at 166 ml/hr. What is the infusion time?

6. It is 11:00 P.M., and 250 ml of fluid remain in an I.V. bag that is infusing at 63 ml/hr. When will the infusion be complete?

7. The nurse must administer 500 ml of Intralipids I.V. at 42 ml/hr. What is the infusion time?

8. The doctor's order states *Infuse 1,150 ml of TPN at 96 ml/hr.* What is the infusion time?

9. A patient needs to receive 3 L of D_5W ½ normal saline at 125 ml/hr. What is the infusion time?

10. A patient is receiving 1 L of TPN over 12 hours. The nurse started the infusion at 10 P.M. How many milliliters of solution should remain in the bag at 3 A.M.?

11. The doctor's order reads, *Fluid challenge of 500 ml of normal saline I.V. at 80 gtt/min.* The nurse prepares for the challenge, using an administration set with a drip factor of 15 gtt/ml. What is the infusion time?

12. A doctor orders 1 unit of whole blood transfused at 33 gtt/min. The total volume of the transfusion is 500 ml; the drip factor is 10 gtt/ml. What is the infusion time? If the transfusion begins at 2:00 P.M., when will it be complete?

13. What is the infusion time for 100 ml of normal saline infused at 50 gtt/min via a microdrip set?

14. A patient must receive 1 unit of fresh frozen plasma at 80 gtt/min. The 1-unit bag contains 220 ml; the drip factor is 10 gtt/ml. What is the infusion time?

15. The nurse must administer 50 ml of antibiotic solution by I.V. piggyback at 30 gtt/min. The drip factor is 10 gtt/ml. What is the infusion time?

Answers to practice problems

◆ *Using the infusion-time formula*

1. 8 hours; 5:00 P.M.

2. 5 hours; 7:00 A.M.

3. 5 hours, 57 minutes

4. 6 hours; 5:00 P.M.

5. 2:18 P.M.

6. nutrient

7. 250 ml

8. 5:00 P.M.

9. seep into

◆ Adapting the infusion-time formula

1. 6 hours, 42 minutes

2. 11 hours, 54 minutes

3. 7 hours, 54 minutes

4. 6 hours, 42 minutes

5. 1 hour

◆ Using the alternative formula method

1. 30 minutes; 9:30 A.M.

2. 13 hours, 54 minutes; 11:54 P.M.

3. 2 hours, 18 minutes

4. 11 hours, 54 minutes

5. 45 minutes

Answers to review problems

1. infusion time

2. total parenteral nutrition (TPN)

3. 2 hours, 12 minutes; 7:12 P.M.

4. 4:12 A.M.

5. 6 hours

6. 3:00 A.M.

7. 11 hours, 54 minutes

8. 12 hours

9. 24 hours

10. 583 ml

11. 1 hour, 34 minutes

12. 2 hours, 30 minutes; 4:30 P.M.

13. 2 hours

14. 27 minutes

15. 17 minutes

Chapter

19

◆

Specialized I.V. Medication Calculations

Sometimes, doctors prescribe medications, such as heparin, aminophylline, and insulin, to be added to large-volume I.V. infusions. These medications may be ordered in milliliters (ml) per hour, milligrams (mg) per hour, or units (U) per hour. To administer them safely, you need to know how to calculate the drug dosage so that it falls within therapeutic limits.

At other times, doctors prescribe large-volume infusions with additives that are designed to maintain or restore electrolyte balance or to supply additional nutrients. In these cases, you must calculate and prepare the correct amount and add it to the solution. This chapter guides you through all of these specialized medication calculations.

Calculating heparin dosages

A common anticoagulant, heparin is used to prevent the formation of new clots and slow the development of preexisting clots. Usually given by the I.V. route, heparin is ordered in doses of U/hr or ml/hr. Each dose is individualized based on the patient's coagulation status, which is measured by the activated partial thromboplastin time (APTT) test.

When heparin is ordered, the nurse must know how to calculate the flow rate accurately and to determine the required units per hour.

Flow rates

The nurse must be able to calculate the flow rate accurately to ensure that the heparin dosage falls within safe and therapeutic limits. This type of calculation differs from the flow rate calculations discussed in Chapter 17 because it is used to administer a drug—not just fluid. To calculate the heparin flow rate, first determine the solution's concentration (U/ml) by dividing the units of drug added to the bag by the milliliters of solution. Then calculate the hourly flow rate.

Patient situations
A medication order states heparin 40,000 U in 1 L of D₅W I.V. Infuse at 1,000 U/hr. *What is the flow rate (ml/hr) of the infusion?*
◆ After converting 1 L to 1,000 ml, set up a proportion with fractions.

$$\frac{1,000 \text{ U}}{\text{X ml}} = \frac{40,000 \text{ U}}{1,000 \text{ ml}}$$

♦ Solve for X.

$$\text{X ml} \times 40{,}000 \text{ U} = 1{,}000 \text{ U} \times 1{,}000 \text{ ml}$$

$$X = \frac{1{,}000 \cancel{U} \times 1{,}000 \text{ ml}}{40{,}000 \cancel{U}}$$

$$X = \frac{1{,}000{,}000 \text{ ml}}{40{,}000}$$

$$X = 25 \text{ ml}$$

To administer heparin at 1,000 U/hour, the nurse should set the flow rate at 25 ml/hour.

The doctor prescribes a continuous infusion of 25,000 U of heparin in 250 ml of D$_5$W. The patient is to receive 600 U/hr. What is the flow rate?

♦ Set up a proportion with ratios.

$$25{,}000 \text{ U} : 250 \text{ ml} :: 600 \text{ U} : \text{X ml}$$

♦ Solve for X.

$$25{,}000 \text{ U} \times \text{X ml} = 250 \text{ ml} \times 600 \text{ U}$$

$$X = \frac{250 \text{ ml} \times 600 \cancel{U}}{25{,}000 \cancel{U}}$$

$$X = \frac{150{,}000 \text{ ml}}{25{,}000}$$

$$X = 6 \text{ ml}$$

To administer 600 U/hr, the nurse should set the flow rate at 6 ml/hr.

Units per hour

If the doctor orders a heparin infusion in ml/hr, the nurse can calculate how many units per hour the patient should receive. This determines the patient's drug dose so the nurse can make sure it falls within a safe and therapeutic range.

Patient situation

A patient is receiving 20,000 U of heparin in 1,000 ml of D$_5$W I.V. at 30 ml/hr. What heparin dose is the patient receiving?

♦ Set up a proportion with fractions.

$$\frac{20{,}000 \text{ U}}{1{,}000 \text{ ml}} = \frac{\text{X U}}{30 \text{ ml}}$$

♦ Solve for X.

$$1{,}000 \text{ ml} \times \text{X U} = 20{,}000 \text{ U} \times 30 \text{ ml}$$

$$X = \frac{20{,}000 \text{ U} \times 30 \cancel{ml}}{1{,}000 \cancel{ml}}$$

$$X = \frac{600{,}000 \text{ U}}{1{,}000}$$

$$X = 600 \text{ U}$$

With the flow rate set at 30 ml/hr, the patient is receiving 600 U/hr.

The nurse can also calculate the heparin dose in units per hour when only the drip rate (gtt/min) and drip factor (gtt/ml) are known.

Calculating heparin dosages

Perform the following calculations related to heparin therapy. To check your answers, see page 216.

1. A patient must receive 1,200 U of heparin per hour. The nurse hangs a bag of 25,000 U of heparin in 250 ml of D₅W. How should the nurse set the flow rate?

2. A patient is receiving 1,500 U of heparin per hour from an I.V. bag that contains 20,000 U of heparin in 500 ml of D₅W. What is the flow rate?

3. The nurse sets up an I.V. infusion of 25,000 U heparin in 250 ml of D₅W, which runs at 16 ml/hr. How many units/hour should the patient receive?

4. A doctor prescribes 20,000 U heparin in 250 ml of D₅W I.V. at 20 ml/hr. How many units per hour should the patient receive?

5. The doctor prescribes 40,000 U heparin in 1 L of D₅W I.V. at 15 gtt/min. The drip factor is 10 gtt/ml. How many units/hour should the nurse administer?

Calculating dosages for continuous insulin infusions

Sometimes, an acutely ill diabetic patient needs to receive insulin by continuous infusion, which allows close control of insulin administration based on serial measurements of the blood glucose level. Regular insulin is the only type that can be administered by the I.V. route, and continuous insulin administration must be performed with an I.V. infusion pump.

Golden Rules

Use only regular insulin when insulin must be administered intravenously.

Usually, the doctor prescribes the dose in units per hour, but can order it in milliliters per hour. No matter how the dose is prescribed, however, the doctor should order the infusion in a concentration of 1 U/ml to avoid calculation errors that can cause serious consequences.

Patient situations

A patient must receive a continuous infusion of 150 U of regular insulin in 150 ml of NS at 6 U/hr. What is the flow rate?

◆ Set up a proportion, using the appropriate information.

$$\frac{150\text{ U}}{150\text{ ml}} = \frac{6\text{ U}}{X\text{ ml}}$$

◆ Solve for X.

$$150 \text{ U} \times X \text{ ml} = 150 \text{ ml} \times 6 \text{ U}$$

$$X = \frac{150 \text{ ml} \times 6 \cancel{U}}{150 \cancel{U}}$$

$$X = \frac{900 \text{ ml}}{150}$$

$$X = 6 \text{ ml}$$

To administer 6 U/hr of the prescribed insulin, the nurse should set the infusion pump's flow rate at 6 ml/hr.

The nurse sets up a continuous infusion of 50 U of regular insulin in 100 ml of NS at 10 ml/hr. How many U/hr is the patient receiving?

◆ Set up a proportion with the given information.

$$\frac{50 \text{ U}}{100 \text{ ml}} = \frac{X \text{ U}}{10 \text{ ml}}$$

◆ Solve for X.

$$100 \text{ ml} \times X \text{ U} = 50 \text{ U} \times 10 \text{ ml}$$

$$X = \frac{50 \text{ U} \times 10 \cancel{ml}}{100 \cancel{ml}}$$

$$X = \frac{500 \text{ U}}{100}$$

$$X = 5 \text{ U}$$

When this insulin infusion runs at 10 ml/hr, the patient is receiving 5 U/hr.

Calculating dosages for continuous insulin infusions

Perform the following calculations related to continuous insulin infusions. To check your answers, see page 216.

1. The nurse starts a continuous infusion of 150 U of regular insulin in 150 ml of NS. The prescribed dose is 8 U/hr. What flow rate delivers this dose?

2. A patient needs to receive a continuous insulin infusion of 12 U/hr. The nurse plans to administer 100 U of regular insulin in 100 ml of NS, as prescribed. What flow rate should the nurse use?

3. An I.V. bag contains 150 U of regular insulin in 150 ml of NS and has been infusing at 4 U/hr. Now, the doctor orders the dose to be increased to 6 U/hr. After the nurse increases the dose, what is the flow rate?

4. An I.V. bag contains 50 U of regular insulin in 50 ml of NS and is infusing at 10 ml/hr. After reviewing the patient's serum glucose level, the doctor orders the dose to be decreased to 8 ml/hr. What is the new dose (in units per hour)?

5. The doctor prescribes an I.V. drip of 50 U of regular insulin in 100 ml of NS, using a flow rate of 20 ml/hr. What is this prescribed dose (in units per hour)?

Calculating dosages of electrolytes and nutrients

I.V. fluids can be used to deliver electrolytes and nutrients directly into the patient's bloodstream. The doctor's order will include the additives to be administered. For example, this order: *D₅W with 20 mEq KCl/L at 100 ml/hr* means that 20 mEq of potassium chloride should be in the liter bag of dextrose 5% in water and that the flow rate for that solution should be 100 ml/hour.

Sometimes, the order calls for more than one additive to be combined in the solution. Before calculating the correct amounts of each substance to inject, check a compatibility chart or consult a pharmacist to ensure that the additives are miscible.

To calculate the amount of additive, use the same equations as for any prepared liquid medication. *Always verify that any additive-containing I.V. solution is labeled with the time, name, and amount of medication added.*

Golden Rules

Always verify that an I.V. solution with additives is labeled with the time, name, and amount of medication added.

Large-volume infusions with additives are administered to maintain or restore hydration or electrolyte status or to supply additional electrolytes, vitamins, or other nutrients. Common additives include potassium chloride, vitamins B and C, and trace elements.

If the additive is not prepackaged in the solution, by the manufacturer or by the facility's pharmacy, the nurse must prepare the correct amount and add it to the solution. Then, as with other I.V. solutions, you must calculate the flow rate and the drip rate.

Patient situations

A patient is to receive 1,000 ml of D₅W with 150 mg of thiamine/L over 12 hours. The thiamine is available in a prepared syringe of 100 mg/ml. How many milliliters of thiamine must be added to the solution?

◆ Using ratios, set up the following proportion.

$$150 \text{ mg} : X \text{ ml} :: 100 \text{ mg} : 1 \text{ ml}$$

◆ Solve for X.

$$X \text{ ml} \times 100 \text{ mg} = 150 \text{ mg} \times 1 \text{ ml}$$

$$X = \frac{150 \text{ ml}}{100}$$

$$X = 1.5 \text{ ml}$$

A doctor's order states **Infuse dextrose 5% in 0.33NS with 40 mEq KCl/L at 80 ml/hr.** *The potassium chloride is available in vials of 20 mEq/10 ml. How many milliliters of potassium chloride should be added to the solution?*

◆ Using fractions, set up the proportion and solve for X.

$$\frac{40 \text{ mEq}}{X \text{ ml}} = \frac{20 \text{ mEq}}{10 \text{ ml}}$$

$$X \text{ ml} \times 20 \text{ mEq} = 40 \text{ mEq} \times 10 \text{ ml}$$

$$X = \frac{400 \text{ ml}}{20}$$

$$X = 20 \text{ ml}$$

◆ Another way to solve this problem would be to determine the strength of each milliliter of the potassium chloride solution. To do so, set up the following proportion and solve for X.

$$\frac{X \text{ mEq}}{1 \text{ ml}} = \frac{20 \text{ mEq}}{10 \text{ ml}}$$

$$X \text{ mEq} \times 10 \text{ ml} = 20 \text{ mEq} \times 1 \text{ ml}$$

$$X = 2 \text{ mEq}$$

◆ Knowing that the available vial contains 2 mEq/ml and that 40 mEq is needed, use the following proportion and solve for X.

$$\frac{40 \text{ mEq}}{X \text{ ml}} = \frac{2 \text{ mEq}}{1 \text{ ml}}$$

$$X \text{ ml} \times 2 \text{ mEq} = 40 \text{ mEq} \times 1 \text{ ml}$$

$$X = \frac{40 \text{ ml}}{2}$$

$$X = 20 \text{ ml}$$

◆ **PRACTICE PROBLEMS**

Calculating dosages of electrolytes and nutrients

Answer the following questions related to electrolyte and nutrient calculations. To check your answers, see page 216.

1. Before calculating the correct amounts of each substance to be injected into an I.V solution, what should the nurse be sure to check?

2. The nurse needs to add 30 mEq of KCl to an I.V. of D5 ½NS. The vial of KCl contains 2 mEq/ml. How many milliliters of KCl should the nurse add to administer the correct dose?

3. A patient needs to receive 100 mg of thiamine in 1 L of normal saline. The thiamine vial contains 100 mg in 5 ml. How many milliliters of thiamine should the nurse add to the I.V. bag?

4. The nurse must add one ampule of calcium gluconate to 1 L of D_5W. One ampule contains 10 ml of the electrolyte. How many milliliters of calcium gluconate should the nurse add to this I.V. fluid?

5. The doctor prescribes 1 L of D_5NS I.V. with 200 mg of ascorbic acid and 60 mEq of KCl. The vial of ascorbic acid contains 100 mg/ml; the vial of KCl contains 2 mEq/ml. How many milliliters of each should the nurse add to the I.V. fluid?

Review problems

Perform the following calculations related to selected I.V. medications. To check your answers, see page 216.

1. A doctor orders 20,000 U of heparin in 500 ml D$_5$W to infuse at 25 ml/hr. How many units of heparin should the patient receive in an hour?

2. A patient is to receive 1,200 U/hour of heparin. Using a solution of 10,000 U of heparin in 250 ml D$_5$W, the nurse should set the infusion pump at what flow rate?

3. A doctor orders 20,000 U of heparin in 500 ml D$_5$W to infuse at 1,500 U/hr. What should the flow rate on the infusion pump be?

4. A patient must receive a solution of 20,000 U of heparin in 500 ml D$_5$W at 34 ml/hr. How many units should the patient receive in 24 hours?

5. A doctor prescribes 20,000 U of heparin in 250 ml D$_5$W to infuse at 16 ml/hr. How many units per hour will the patient receive?

6. What type of insulin can be administered by I.V. infusion?

7. A patient must receive a continuous infusion of 150 U of insulin in 150 ml of normal saline. The nurse sets the flow rate at 11 ml/hr. How many units per hour should the patient receive?

8. The nurse adds 100 U of insulin to 50 ml of normal saline and then infuses it at 12 U/hr. How many milliliters per hour should be infused?

9. The doctor's order reads *Insulin 150 U in 150 ml of normal saline I.V. to run at 14 ml/hr.* What is the dose in units per hour?

10. The nurse starts an infusion of 100 U of insulin in 100 ml of normal saline to run at 2 U/hr. After reviewing the patient's blood glucose level, the doctor orders the infusion rate to be increased to 5 U/hr. After the nurse increases the dose, what should the flow rate be?

11. A doctor's order states: *3 L dextrose 5% in ½NS in 24 hours. Add 1 vial M.V.I.-12 to first L.* Each vial of M.V.I.-12 contains 5 ml. How many milliliters should the nurse add to the first liter of I.V. fluid?

12. A patient is to receive 20 mEq of KCl/L of I.V. fluid. The vial states that there are 2 mEq/ml. How many milliliters of KCl should the nurse add?

13. A patient must receive 50 mg of thiamine in 1 L of dextrose 5% in ⅓NS. The thiamine vial contains 100 mg in 5 ml. How many milliliters of thiamine should the nurse add to the I.V. solution?

14. A doctor orders one vial of vitamin B complex with vitamin C and an ampule of trace elements to be added to the patient's I.V. fluids. The vial of vitamin B complex with vitamin C contains 5 ml. The ampule of trace elements contains 2 ml. How many milliliters of vitamin B complex with vitamin C should the nurse add to the I.V. bottle? How many milliliters of trace elements?

15. A hypokalemic patient needs to receive 40 mEq of KCl in 500 ml of dextrose 5% in ½NS to infuse over 4 hours. The KCl vial contains 2 mEq/ml. How many milliliters of KCl should the nurse add to the I.V. solution?

Answers to practice problems

◆ **Calculating heparin dosages**

1. 12 ml/hr
2. 37.5 ml/hr
3. 1,600 U/hr
4. 1,600 U/hr
5. 3,600 U/hr

◆ **Calculating dosages for continuous insulin infusions**

1. 8 ml/hr
2. 12 ml/hr
3. 6 ml/hr
4. 8 U/hr
5. 10 U/hr

◆ **Calculating dosages of electrolytes and nutrients**

1. compatibility
2. 15 ml
3. 5 ml
4. 10 ml
5. 2 ml of ascorbic acid; 30 ml of KCl

Answers to review problems

1. 1,000 U/hr
2. 30 ml/hr
3. 37.5 or 38 ml/hr
4. 32,640 U
5. 1,280 U/hr
6. regular insulin
7. 11 U/hr
8. 6 ml/hr
9. 14 U/hr
10. 5 ml/hr
11. 5 ml
12. 10 ml
14. 2.5 ml
14. 5 ml of vitamins; 2 ml of trace elements
15. 20 ml

UNIT 6

◆

Special Dosage Calculations

Unit 6 presents special dosage calculations that the nurse may use when caring for pediatric, obstetric, or critically ill patients. Many of the drugs used for these patients have a small margin for error. Because of this, the nurse must take extra care with dosage calculations to ensure their accuracy in all of these specialty areas.

Chapter 20 describes how pediatric patients differ from adult patients. It covers methods for calculating pediatric dosages, including those based on weight and body surface area. It also provides guidelines for administering I.V. fluids to pediatric patients and for calculating their fluid needs.

Chapter 21 discusses the complexity of caring for obstetric patients. It also walks through the steps needed to calculate dosages of drugs that are unique to obstetrics.

Chapter 22 introduces drugs for critical care. These drugs must be administered rapidly and accurately to save patients' lives. The chapter demonstrates how to calculate dosages for drugs given by I.V. push and I.V. infusion.

Chapter

20

◆
Pediatric Dosages

Caring for pediatric patients presents challenges related to their developmental stage. That is why their drug dosages may need to be individualized and their administration modified.

This chapter shows how to do pediatric dosage calculations based on the body weight and body surface area. It also demonstrates methods for calculating fluid needs based on age and weight. Because children's bodies allow only a small margin for error, the nurse must ensure that pediatric dosage and fluid calculations are accurate.

Pediatric patients and drugs

When caring for a pediatric patient, remember that a child is not simply a small adult. Although drug administration routes are the same for children and adults, safe dosage ranges can differ greatly. Pediatric dosages differ from those for adults because a child's immature body systems may be unable to handle certain drugs. For example, a child's volume of total body water is much higher than an adult's, and this affects drug distribution. The pharmacokinetics, pharmacodynamics, and pharmacotherapeutics of drugs differ in children, requiring special dosages.

Drug preparation and administration also may differ for children. For example, oral medications are prepared as liquids for infants and young children who cannot swallow tablets or capsules. When a liquid preparation is not available and the child must receive a tablet, the nurse may crush and administer it with a small amount of liquid. However, the nurse must *not* crush time-release capsules or tablets or enteric-coated medications. Crushing destroys the coating, which allows drug release at the appropriate time.

The nurse can measure and administer liquid medications in a medication cup that provides measurements in the metric and household systems. If the child is very young and cannot drink from a cup, the nurse can use a medication dropper. (Droppers are sometimes packaged with medications.)

If the liquid medication is prepared as a suspension (an insoluble drug in a liquid base), the nurse must mix the suspension thoroughly before measuring and administering it to ensure that none of the medication has settled out of the solution. Whenever an oral medication is administered, the nurse must make sure that the child has swallowed it by inspecting the child's mouth.

In addition to oral medications, pediatric patients may receive parenteral medications. Drugs administered by the subcutaneous (S.C.) route include insulin and childhood immunizations.

Because of its subcutaneous tissue, the upper arm is the most common site for such immunizations, but any area with sufficient subcutaneous tissue is acceptable.

Drugs commonly administered by the intramuscular (I.M.) route include diphtheria, pertussis, and tetanus (DPT) vaccine and medications for pain and sedation. The nurse should ensure that each I.M. injection contains no more than 1 ml of solution. Also, the nurse should administer I.M. injections in the thigh for infants and young children because the gluteal muscles do not develop until the child has learned to walk.

Fluids and drugs may be administered by the intravenous (I.V.) route. Because pediatric patients can tolerate only a narrow range of fluid, the nurse should dilute I.V. drugs carefully and administer I.V. fluids cautiously. Also, the nurse should inspect I.V. sites frequently for signs of infiltration or inflammation because children's vessels are immature and easily damaged by drugs.

Pediatric patients and drugs

Answer the following questions about pediatric patients and drugs. To check your answers, see page 234.

1. Drug administration routes are _____ in children and adults.
2. If a young child cannot drink from a cup, the nurse can use a _____ _____ to administer a liquid medication.
3. A drug in suspension form must be _____ thoroughly before it is measured and administered.
4. Insulin and childhood _____ are administered by the S.C. route.
5. For a child, an I.M. injection should contain no more than _____ of solution.

Calculating pediatric dosages

To calculate pediatric drug dosages accurately, use the dosage per kilogram of body weight or body surface area (BSA) method. (See *Using a BSA nomogram*, page 223, for details.) Other methods, based on the child's weight or age, are less accurate but may be used for rough estimates. Whichever method is used, the nurse is professionally and legally responsible for checking the prescribed pediatric dosage to ensure that it falls within the safe dosage range.

Dosage per kilogram of body weight

Many pharmaceutical companies provide information about safe drug dosages for pediatric patients in milligrams per kilogram of body weight. Based on this information, the nurse can determine the pediatric dosage by multiplying the child's body weight in kilograms by the milligrams of drug per kilogram. Most nurses consider this the most accurate method of determining pediatric drug dosages.

Converting to kilograms

Because most patients are measured in pounds, the nurse must be able to convert from pounds to kilograms before calculating the dosage per kilogram of body weight.

Patient situation

The doctor prescribes furosemide (Lasix) 1 mg/kg I.V. for a child who weighs 45 lb. Determine the child's weight in kilograms.

◆ Set up the proportion. Remember that 2.2 lb is the equivalent of 1 kg.

$$X \text{ kg} : 45 \text{ lb} :: 1 \text{ kg} : 2.2 \text{ lb}$$

◆ Solve for X.

$$X \text{ kg} \times 2.2 \text{ lb} = 45 \text{ lb} \times 1 \text{ kg}$$

$$X = \frac{45 \text{ lb} \times 1 \text{ kg}}{2.2 \text{ lb}}$$

$$X = 20.45 \text{ or } 20.5 \text{ kg}$$

The child weighs 20 kg.

Calculating dosages

Once the pediatric patient's weight in kilograms has been determined, the nurse can use this information to calculate an individualized drug dosage.

Patient situations

If the suggested pediatric dosage for a drug is 30 mg/kg/day, use the dosage per kilogram of body weight method to calculate how much drug to give an infant who weighs 7 kg.

◆ Set up a proportion with the suggested dosage in one ratio and the unknown quantity in the second ratio.

$$30 \text{ mg} : 1 \text{ kg} :: X \text{ mg} : 7 \text{ kg}$$

◆ Solve for X.

$$X \text{ mg} \times 1 \text{ kg} = 30 \text{ mg} \times 7 \text{ kg}$$

$$X = \frac{30 \text{ mg} \times 7 \text{ kg}}{1 \text{ kg}}$$

$$X = 210 \text{ mg}$$

A pediatrician orders propylthiouracil (PTU) 10 mg/kg/day P.O. in divided doses to be given every 8 hours. The drug is available in 50-mg tablets and the child weighs 67 lb. What volume of drug should the nurse administer at each dose?

◆ Determine the child's weight in kilograms using the conversion factor 1 kg = 2.2 lb and ratios in a proportion.

$$X \text{ kg} : 67 \text{ lb} :: 1 \text{ kg} : 2.2 \text{ lb}$$

◆ Solve for X.

$$X \text{ kg} \times 2.2 \text{ lb} = 67 \text{ lb} \times 1 \text{ kg}$$

$$X = \frac{67 \text{ kg}}{2.2}$$

$$X = 30.45, \text{ or } 30.5 \text{ kg}$$

◆ Because the child is to receive 10 mg/kg, use the following proportion with fractions to determine the total loading dose.

$$\frac{30.5 \text{ kg}}{X \text{ mg}} = \frac{1 \text{ kg}}{10 \text{ mg}}$$

◆ Solve for X.

$$X \text{ mg} \times 1 \text{ kg} = 30.5 \text{ kg} \times 10 \text{ mg}$$
$$X = 305 \text{ mg}$$

The child's daily dosage is 305 mg.

◆ Divide the daily dosage by 3 to determine the dose to administer every 8 hours.

$$X = \frac{305 \text{ mg}}{3}$$
$$X = 101.7, \text{ or } 102 \text{ mg}$$

The child should receive 102 mg for each dose.

◆ Find the number of tablets to give at each dose by setting up a proportion and solving for X.

$$\frac{X \text{ tab}}{102 \text{ mg}} = \frac{1 \text{ tab}}{50 \text{ mg}}$$
$$X \text{ tab} \times 50 \text{ mg} = 102 \text{ mg} \times 1 \text{ tab}$$
$$X = \frac{102 \text{ tab}}{50}$$
$$X = 2.04, \text{ or } 2 \text{ tablets}$$

Administer 2 tablets of the drug at each dose.

A 44-lb child must receive streptomycin sulfate, 30 mg/kg/day in divided doses every 12 hours. The drug is available in 1-g vials that can be diluted to produce 1 g/3 ml. What volume of drug should the nurse administer at each dose?

◆ Determine the child's weight in kilograms using ratios in a proportion.

$$X \text{ kg} : 44 \text{ lb} :: 1 \text{ kg} : 2.2 \text{ lb}$$

◆ Solve for X.

$$X \text{ kg} \times 2.2 \text{ lb} = 44 \text{ lb} \times 1 \text{ kg}$$
$$X = \frac{44 \text{ kg}}{2.2}$$
$$X = 20 \text{ kg}$$

◆ Calculate the amount of medication to administer daily by setting up a proportion with the divided dose per kilogram in one ratio and the unknown quantity in the other.

$$X \text{ mg} : 20 \text{ kg} :: 30 \text{ mg} : 1 \text{ kg}$$

◆ Solve for X.

$$X \text{ mg} \times 1 \text{ kg} = 20 \text{ kg} \times 30 \text{ mg}$$
$$X = 600 \text{ mg}$$

The child should receive a total daily dosage of 600 mg.

◆ Divide the total dosage by 2 to determine the dose to administer every 12 hours.

$$X = \frac{600 \text{ mg}}{2}$$
$$X = 300 \text{ mg}$$

The child should receive 300 mg, or 0.3 g, for each dose.

◆ Set up a proportion to determine the volume of drug to give at each dose.

$$X \text{ ml} : 0.3 \text{ g} :: 3 \text{ ml} : 1 \text{ g}$$

♦ Solve for X.

$$X \text{ ml} \times 1 \text{ g} = 0.3 \text{ g} \times 3 \text{ ml}$$
$$X = 0.9 \text{ ml}$$

Administer 0.9 ml of streptomycin sulfate at each dose.

Dosages by BSA

An accurate way to calculate safe pediatric dosages is by BSA. This is a two-step process. First, the nurse determines the patient's BSA. Then, the nurse multiplies the BSA by the pediatric dosage (in milligrams per square meter).

Determining BSA

To determine BSA in square meters (m²), the nurse plots the patient's height and weight on a nomogram. (See *Using a BSA nomogram* for details.)

Patient situation

An infant weighs 7 lb and is 19" long. Determine the infant's BSA.
♦ First locate the infant's height (length) in the left column and his weight in the right column of the BSA nomogram.
♦ Using a ruler, draw a straight line connecting the two points. Note that the line intersects the middle column at 0.21, indicating that the infant's BSA is 0.21 m².
♦ As an alternative for an average-size child, use a single-column nomogram. Simply find the child's weight in pounds on the left side of the scale. Then read the corresponding BSA on the right side.

Calculating dosages

After finding the pediatric patient's BSA in square meters, the nurse can calculate the dosage by multiplying the prescribed dosage (in milligrams per square meter) times the BSA. The following equation shows how.

$$\text{m}^2 \text{ (child's BSA)} \times \frac{(\text{drug dose}) \text{ mg}}{1 \text{ m}^2} = \text{child's dose}$$

This calculation method usually is used to calculate safe adult and pediatric dosages for antineoplastic drugs, such as methotrexate and cytarabine.

When the nurse needs to calculate an approximate pediatric dose based on an adult dose, the BSA method can help ensure accuracy. Use the child's BSA in the following equation.

$$\text{child's dose} = \frac{\text{child's BSA}}{\text{average adult BSA (1.73 m}^2)} \times \text{average adult dose}$$

Patient situations

The suggested pediatric dosage for ephedrine (Ephed II) is 100 mg/m²/day. If a child is 40" tall and weighs 64 lb, how much ephedrine should the child receive daily?
♦ Use the nomogram to determine that the BSA is 0.92 m².
♦ Determine the daily dosage using fractions in a proportion.

$$\frac{X \text{ mg}}{0.92 \text{ m}^2} = \frac{100 \text{ mg}}{1 \text{ m}^2}$$
$$X \text{ mg} \times 1 \text{ m}^2 = 0.92 \text{ m}^2 \times 100 \text{ mg}$$
$$X = 92 \text{ mg}$$

Using a BSA nomogram

When calculating the dosage of an extremely potent drug (or of a drug for a pediatric patient), first determine the patient's body surface area (BSA). To do this, plot the patient's height and weight on the nomogram, and connect these two points with a straight line. The point where this line intersects the BSA scale is the patient's BSA in square meters (m²). For example, suppose a patient is 160 cm tall and weighs 65 kg. A straight line connecting the height and weight intersects the middle scale at 1.75, indicating that the patient's BSA is 1.75 m².

For an average-size child, use the simplified nomogram, below right. This scale determines BSA based on the patient's weight alone.

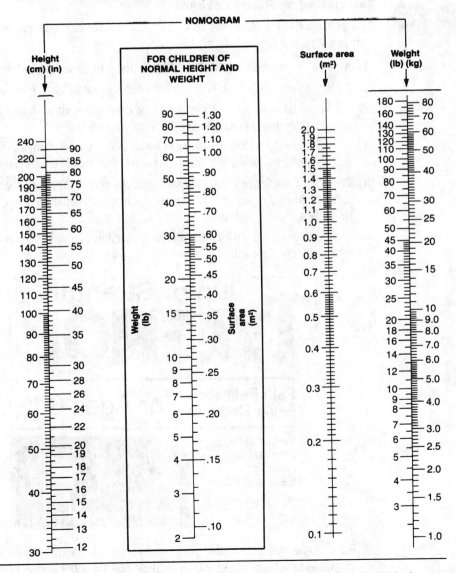

Reprinted with permission from Richard E. Behrman ed. *Nelson Textbook of Pediatrics,* 15th ed. Philadelphia: W.B. Saunders Co., 1996.

A child is 36" tall and weighs 40 lb. What would be a safe dose for this child if the average adult dose is 1 g (1,000 mg)?

◆ Use the nomogram to determine that the child's BSA is 0.70 m².

◆ Divide the child's BSA by 1.73 m² (the average adult BSA), and multiply the result by the average adult dose.

$$X = \frac{0.70 \text{ m}^2}{1.73 \text{ m}^2} \times 1{,}000 \text{ mg}$$

$$X = \frac{700 \text{ mg}}{1.73}$$

$$X = 404.6 \text{ or } 405 \text{ mg}$$

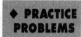

Calculating pediatric dosages

Answer the following questions about pediatric dosage calculations. To check your answers, see pages 234 and 235.

1. A pediatric patient weighs 67 lb. What is this child's weight in kilograms?

2. An infant weighs 9 lb, 3 oz. How much does this infant weigh in kilograms?

3. A 30-lb child must receive 10 mg/kg of a drug, three times a day. How many milligrams should the child receive with each dose?

4. A child who weighs 75 lb needs to receive a loading dose of phenytoin (Dilantin), 15 mg/kg I.V. How many milligrams of the drug should the child receive?

5. The doctor's order reads *Administer erythromycin stearate 30 mg/kg P.O. daily in divided doses q6h.* How many milligrams should an 18-kg pediatric patient receive with each dose?

6. A child who weighs 30 kg is to receive ampicillin 50 mg/kg/day. What is total daily dosage for this patient?

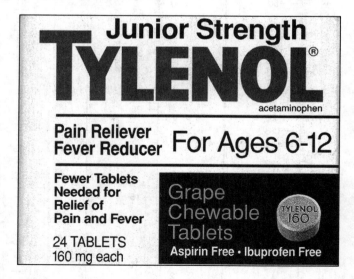

7. For a febrile pediatric patient who weighs 40 lb, the doctor orders Tylenol chewable tablets 10 mg/kg P.O. q4h. Based on the label above, how many tablets should this patient receive?

8. A child is 94 cm tall and weighs 16 kg. What is the child's BSA?

9. A pediatric patient weighs 50 lb and is 40″ tall. What is this patient's BSA?

10. A pediatric patient who needs chemotherapy weighs 100 lb and is 60″ tall. What is this patient's BSA?

11. The suggested pediatric dosage for chlorambucil (Leukeran) is 4.5 mg/m²/day. If a child is 45″ tall and weighs 70 lb, how much chlorambucil should the child receive daily?

12. A patient with a BSA of 1.1 m² needs to receive cyclophosphamide 250 mg/m² P.O. daily for 6 days. What is the daily dose for this patient?

13. A pediatric patient with leukemia has a BSA of 0.8 m² and must receive a daily dose of mercaptopurine 75 mg/m² (rounded to the nearest 25 mg) P.O. The drug is supplied in 50-mg tablets. How many tablets should the patient receive?

14. A child with a urinary tract infection has a BSA of 0.9 m². For this patient, the doctor prescribes sulfisoxazole (Gantrisin) 2 g/m² P.O. daily in divided doses q6h. The drug comes in liquid form with a dosage strength of 500 mg/5 ml. How many milliliters should the child receive in each dose?

Other calculations for pediatric dosages

To verify pediatric dosages, the nurse can use one of three other calculations: Fried's rule, Clark's rule, or Young's rule. Because these rules derive the pediatric dosage from an average adult dosage and assume an average developmental level for a child, their results are only approximate. They can be used to help verify dosages, *not* to determine them.

Fried's rule

Based on the child's age only, Fried's rule usually is used to verify dosages for infants under age 1.

$$\frac{\text{child's age (months)}}{\substack{\text{150 months (age at which an} \\ \text{adult dose would be appropriate)}}} \times \text{average adult dose} = \text{child's dose}$$

Patient situation

The average adult dose of a drug is 500 mg. The nurse needs to determine the size of the dose for a 6-month-old child.

$$\frac{6 \text{ months}}{150 \text{ months}} \times 500 \text{ mg} = 20 \text{ mg (child's dose)}$$

Clark's rule

Based on body weight only, Clark's rule should be used for children over age 2. With this rule, the younger the child, the less accurate the dosage.

$$\frac{\text{child's weight (lb)}}{150 \text{ lb (average adult weight)}} \times \text{average adult dose} = \text{child's dose}$$

Patient situation

The average adult dose of cefoperazone (Cefobid) is 1 g (1,000 mg). The nurse must determine how much drug to administer to an 8-year-old who weighs 76 lb.

$$\frac{76 \text{ lb}}{150 \text{ lb}} \times 1{,}000 \text{ mg} = 506.67, \text{ or } 507 \text{ mg (child's dose)}$$

Young's rule

Based on the child's age only, Young's rule usually is used for children ages 2 to 12.

$$\frac{\text{child's age (yr)}}{\text{child's age (yr)} + 12} \times \text{average adult dose} = \text{child's dose}$$

Patient situation

The average adult dose of penicillin V potassium is 250 mg. The nurse must determine how many milligrams to give to a child age 8.

$$\frac{8 \text{ yr}}{8 \text{ yr} + 12 \text{ yr}} \times 250 \text{ mg} = 100 \text{ mg (child's dose)}$$

Dosage range calculations

Besides using Fried's, Clark's, or Young's rule, the nurse can use drug-label or package-insert information to verify pediatric dosages. To do this, the nurse finds the safe dosage range on the drug information, calculates the low and high dosages, and determines if the prescribed dosage falls in that range.

Patient situation

The doctor's order states cefaclor (Ceclor) 200 mg P.O. daily in divided doses t.i.d. The pediatric patient weighs 25 kg. Is the prescribed dosage safe for this patient?
◆ First, check the drug label for dosage information.

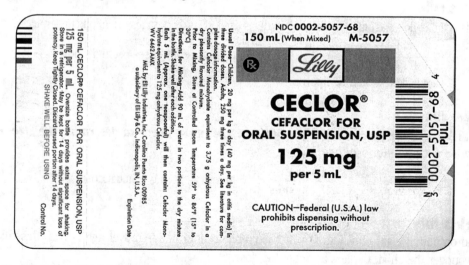

Based on the label information, the nurse knows that the usual pediatric dosage is 20 mg/kg a day (or 40 mg/kg in otitis media) in three divided doses. So the low dose is 20 mg/kg/day; the high dose, 40 mg/kg/day.

◆ Next, calculate the low and high dosages for a patient who weighs 25 kg.

Low dosage = 20 mg × 25 kg = 500 mg/day

High dosage = 40 mg × 25 kg = 1,000 mg/day

Therefore, the recommended dosage range is 500 to 1,000 mg/day for a 25-kg child.

◆ Then, because the daily dosage must be administered in three divided doses, calculate the range for each individual dose.

$$\text{Low dosage} = \frac{500 \text{ mg}}{3 \text{ doses}} = 166.6 \text{ or } 167 \text{ mg per dose}$$

$$\text{High dosage} = \frac{1,000 \text{ mg}}{3 \text{ doses}} = 333.3 \text{ or } 333 \text{ mg per dose}$$

◆ Finally, compare the doctor's order against the safe range of 167 to 333 mg per dose for a 25-kg child. Since the doctor ordered 200 mg per dose, this amount is safe to administer.

If the prescribed amount falls above — or below — the safe dosage range, consult with the doctor to review and revise the drug order as needed. Remember: Doses that are too high may cause adverse effects, but doses that are too low may delay recovery.

Other calculations for pediatric dosages

Answer the following questions about pediatric dosage calculations. To check your answers, see page 235.

1. Using Fried's rule, calculate the pediatric dosages for these problems.

   a) If the average adult dose of ipecac syrup is 30 ml, how many milliliters should the nurse give to an infant age 11 months?

   b) If the average adult dose of hydroxyzine (Vistaril) syrup is 50 mg, how many milligrams should the nurse give to an 8-month-old infant?

2. Using Clark's rule, calculate the pediatric dosages for these problems.

   a) If the average adult dose of furosemide (Lasix) injection is 40 mg, how many milligrams should a 30-lb child receive?

   b) If the average adult dose of digoxin (Lanoxin) is 0.25 mg (250 mcg), how many micrograms should the nurse give to a 53-lb child?

3. Using Young's rule, calculate the pediatric dosages for these problems.

   a) If the average adult dose of clindamycin (Cleocin) injection is 600 mg, how many milligrams should the nurse give to a child age 9?

   b) If the average adult dose of meperidine (Demerol) is 0.075 g, how many milligrams should the nurse administer to a child age 11?

4. Based on the following situation, answer the questions below. The doctor prescribes erythromycin 300 mg I.V. q6h for a 40-kg child. The nurse notes that the recommended dosage range is 15 to 20 mg/kg I.V. daily in divided doses every 6 hours.

   a) What is the low recommended dosage? How many milligrams should be in each dose?

   b) What is the high recommended dosage? How many milligrams should be in each dose?

   c) Does the prescribed dosage fall within the recommended range?

5. An infant who weighs 4 kg must receive penicillin V potassium, 35 mg I.V. every 4 hours. According to the package insert, the recommended dosage range is 15 to 56 mg/kg daily in six divided doses. Does the prescribed dosage fall within the recommended range?

Following pediatric guidelines and protocols

Because of the complexity of pediatric I.V. medication administration, the nurse should follow all guidelines and protocols about dosages, fluid volumes for dilution, and administration rates. The nurse can administer I.V. medications by continuous or intermittent infusion.

Guidelines for continuous infusions

To prepare for a continuous infusion, the nurse must add the medication to a small-volume bag of I.V. fluid. When doing this, carefully follow all guidelines for mixing the solution, and remember that pediatric patients can tolerate only small amounts of fluid.

Begin by calculating the dosage and drawing up the drug in a syringe. Next, using aseptic technique, add the drug to the I.V. bag using the drug additive port. Mix the drug thoroughly. Label the I.V. bag with the drug, dosage, time and date it was mixed, and your initials as the person who prepared the solution. Hang the solution and administer the drug by infusion pump at the prescribed flow rate.

Guidelines for intermittent infusions

Drugs administered by intermittent infusion usually are infused with a volume control device, such as a Buretrol, Soluset, or Voluset. (They also can be infused from small-volume bags of I.V. fluid with a microdrip set.) Volume control devices have a 100- to 150-ml fluid chamber, which is calibrated in 1-ml increments to allow accurate fluid administration. Accuracy is especially important with pediatric patients because they cannot tolerate as much fluid as adults and, consequently, can develop fluid overload more easily.

When a volume control device is used, follow the facility's guidelines. Add the prescribed volume of I.V. fluid (which serves as the diluent) to the fluid chamber. Depending on facility policy, consider the drug volume as part of the diluent volume. For example, if 100 mg of a drug is contained in 5 ml of fluid and the total fluid volume should be 50 ml, add 45 ml of diluent because 45 ml (diluent) + 5 ml (drug volume) totals 50 ml. Some facilities do *not* include the drug volume in the total diluent volume so it is important to know your facility's policy.

After careful calculation, draw up the prescribed volume of the drug. Using aseptic technique, add the drug to the fluid chamber through the drug additive port. Mix the drug thoroughly. Then, attach the volume control device to an electronic controller or infusion pump to control the infusion rate. If the I.V. system has a small-volume I.V. bag instead of a volume control device and pump, use a microdrip set, which has a drip factor of 60 gtt/ml. Calculate the appropriate flow rate and infuse the drug. Label the volume control device with the name of the drug being infused.

When the infusion is complete, flush the line to clear the tubing of medication. For a peripheral line, the standard flush is 15 ml; for a central line, it is 20 ml. Administer the flush at the same rate as the medication. Label the volume control device to indicate that the flush is infusing. When the flush is complete, disconnect the device. Remember to assess the I.V. site frequently during the infusion because children's veins are immature and fragile.

Dosage protocols

Drug dosage protocols are safety measures designed to help the nurse ensure that pediatric patients receive correct drug dosages. They provide a recommended dosage range so the nurse can check the prescribed dosage against the recommended one. Any one of the dosage range calculations discussed above can be used.

◆ PRACTICE PROBLEMS

Following pediatric guidelines and protocols

Answer the following questions about pediatric guidelines and protocols. To check your answers, see page 235.

1. The nurse must flush an I.V. line after an intermittent infusion of an I.V. medication. How much fluid should the nurse use to flush a peripheral line? A central line?

2. For an infusion that totals 25 ml, the nurse must add 2 ml of a drug. How much diluent should the nurse add to the fluid chamber if policy states, "Include the drug volume as part of the total infusion volume"?

3. The doctor prescribes ephedrine sulfate (Ephed II) 140 mg I.V. daily, in four divided doses for a 35-kg hypotensive child. The recommended dosage for the drug is 3 mg/kg daily. Does the prescribed dosage fall in the recommended range?

4. To administer drugs by intermittent infusion from small-volume bags of I.V. fluid, the nurse should use a _____ set.

5. If a medication is infused at 60 gtt/min, what infusion rate should the nurse use to flush the line?

Calculating pediatric fluid needs

Infants and children have a greater need than adults for water and are more vulnerable to alterations in fluid and electrolyte balance. Because of the increased percentage of water in their extracellular fluid, children have a fluid exchange rate two to three times higher than that of adults and are, therefore, more susceptible to dehydration. Thus, determining and meeting the fluid needs of children is an important nursing responsibility. The nurse can calculate the number of milliliters of fluid a child requires based on weight in kilograms, metabolism (calories required), BSA in square meters, or age. Although results may vary slightly depending on the method used, all these methods are appropriate. (Note, however, that calculating fluid needs based on age is the least preferable method, because of the variability of size for any particular age.)

This section explains each method for calculating fluid needs of children. Note that fluid replacement can be affected by clinical conditions that result in fluid retention or loss. Children with these conditions receive fluids based on their particular needs.

Calculating fluid needs based on weight

A child who weighs less than 10 kg requires 100 ml of fluid for every kilogram of body weight. To determine this child's fluid needs, follow these steps.

◆ Convert the child's weight in pounds to kilograms.

$$\frac{\text{weight (lb)}}{2.2} = \text{weight (kg)}$$

♦ Multiply the result by 100 ml/kg.

$$\text{weight (kg)} \times 100 \text{ ml/kg} = \text{fluid requirements (ml/day)}$$

A child weighing 10 to 20 kg requires 1,000 ml of fluid for the first 10 kg plus 50 ml for every kilogram above 10. To determine this child's fluid needs, follow these steps.

♦ Convert the child's weight in pounds to kilograms, using the equation above.

♦ Assign 1,000 ml of fluid to the first 10 kg.

♦ Subtract 10 kg from the child's total weight, and multiply the remainder by 50 ml/kg.

$$(\text{total kg} - 10 \text{ kg}) \times 50 \text{ ml/kg} = \text{additional fluids needed}$$

♦ Add this result to the base 1,000 ml. The total is the child's daily fluid requirement.

$$1,000 \text{ ml} + \text{additional fluids needed} = \text{fluid requirements (ml/day)}$$

A child weighing more than 20 kg requires 1,500 ml of fluid for the first 20 kg plus 20 ml for every kilogram above 20. To determine this child's fluid needs, follow these steps.

♦ Convert the child's weight in pounds to kilograms, using the equation above.

♦ Assign 1,500 ml of fluid to the first 20 kg.

♦ Subtract 20 kg from the child's total weight, and multiply the remainder by 20 ml/kg.

$$(\text{total kg} - 20 \text{ kg}) \times 20 \text{ ml/kg} = \text{additional fluids needed}$$

♦ Add this result to the base 1,500 ml. The total is the child's daily fluid requirement.

$$1,500 \text{ ml} + \text{additional fluids needed} = \text{fluid requirements (ml/day)}$$

Calculating fluid needs based on calories of metabolism

The nurse also can calculate fluid needs based on a child's caloric needs, because water is necessary to metabolize calories. A child should receive 120 ml of fluid for every 100 kcal (kilocalories) of metabolism. To calculate the fluid requirements, first find the child's calorie requirement. Calorie requirements can be determined from tables of recommended dietary allowances for children or can be calculated by a dietitian. Next, divide the calorie requirements by 100 (because the fluid requirements have been determined for every 100 cal). Then multiply the result by 120 ml (the amount of fluid required for every 100 kcal), as shown in this equation.

$$\frac{\text{calorie requirements}}{100} \times 120 \text{ ml/kcal} = \text{fluid requirements (ml/day)}$$

Calculating fluid needs based on BSA

Another method for determining pediatric maintenance fluid requirements is based on the child's BSA. To determine the daily fluid needs of a child who is not dehydrated, multiply the child's BSA by 1,500, as shown in this equation.

$$\text{BSA (m}^2\text{)} \times 1,500 \text{ ml/day/m}^2 = \text{maintenance fluid requirements (ml/day)}$$

Calculating fluid needs based on age

A child under age 1 requires 125 to 150 ml per kilogram.

♦ To determine the lower boundary for the range of fluid needed, multiply the child's weight by 125 ml/kg.

$$\text{weight (kg)} \times 125 \text{ ml/kg} = \text{lower boundary (ml/day)}$$

♦ To determine the upper boundary of the range, multiply the child's weight by 150 ml/kg.

$$\text{weight (kg)} \times 150 \text{ ml/kg} = \text{upper boundary (ml/day)}$$

A child age 1 or older requires an initial 1,000 ml of fluid plus 100 ml for each year above 1 (not to exceed 2,500 ml/day). To determine the fluid needs of this child, follow these steps.

◆ Assign 1,000 ml of fluid for the first year.

◆ Subtract 1 year from the child's age, and multiply the remainder by 100 ml.

$$(Age - 1 \text{ year}) \times 100 \text{ ml} = \text{additional fluids needed}$$

◆ Add the result to the base 1,000 ml. The total is the child's daily fluid requirement.

$$1,000 \text{ ml} + \text{additional fluids needed} = \text{fluid requirements (ml/day)}$$

Patient situations

A child weighs 40 lb. How much fluid should the nurse give over 24 hours to meet this child's maintenance needs?

◆ Determine the child's weight in kilograms.

$$\frac{40 \text{ lb}}{X \text{ kg}} = \frac{2.2 \text{ lb}}{1 \text{ kg}}$$

$$X = \frac{40 \text{ kg}}{2.2}$$

$$X = 18.2 \text{ kg}$$

◆ Assign 1,000 ml of fluid for the first 10 kg.

◆ Subtract 10 kg from the child's weight, and multiply the remainder by 50 ml/kg.

$$X = (18.2 \text{ kg} - 10 \text{ kg}) \times 50 \text{ ml/kg}$$

$$X = 8.2 \times 50$$

$$X = 410 \text{ ml}$$

◆ Add the result to the base 1,000 ml.

$$X = 1,000 \text{ ml} + 410 \text{ ml}$$

$$X = 1,410 \text{ ml}$$

A pediatric patient uses 900 calories per day. What are the child's daily fluid requirements?

◆ Set up the equation and solve for X.

$$X = \frac{900 \text{ kcal}}{100} \times 120 \text{ ml/kcal}$$

$$X = 9 \text{ kcal} \times 120 \text{ ml/kcal}$$

$$X = 1,080 \text{ ml}$$

An infant has a BSA of 0.25 m². How much fluid does the infant require each day?

◆ Set up the following equation and solve for X.

$$X = 0.25 \times 1,500 \text{ ml/day}$$

$$X = 375 \text{ ml/day}$$

A pediatric patient has a BSA of about 1.57 m². How much fluid does the patient require each day?

◆ Set up the following equation and solve for X.

$$X = 1.57 \times 1,500 \text{ ml/day}$$
$$X = 2,355 \text{ ml/day}$$

Thus, the child should receive 2,355 ml of fluid each day.

If the patient is 4½ years old, how much fluid does the child require each day?

◆ Assign an initial 1,000 ml of fluid for the first year.

◆ Subtract 1 year from the patient's age, and multiply the remainder by 100 ml.

$$X = (4.5 - 1) \times 100 \text{ ml}$$
$$X = 3.5 \times 100 \text{ ml}$$
$$X = 350 \text{ ml}$$

◆ Add the result to the base 1,000 ml.

$$X = 1,000 \text{ ml} + 350 \text{ ml}$$
$$X = 1,350 \text{ ml}$$

What is the appropriate range of fluid volume that the nurse should administer to a child age 5 months who weighs 6 kg?

◆ To determine the lower boundary for the range of fluid that the patient should receive, set up the following equation and solve for X.

$$X = 6 \text{ kg} \times 125 \text{ ml/kg}$$
$$X = 750 \text{ ml}$$

◆ To determine the upper boundary for the amount of fluid that the patient should receive, set up the following equation and solve for X.

$$X = 6 \text{ kg} \times 150 \text{ ml/kg}$$
$$X = 900 \text{ ml}$$

The patient should receive 750 to 900 ml of fluid to meet maintenance fluid needs.

Calculating pediatric fluid needs

Calculate the pediatric fluid needs in the following problems. To check your answers, see page 235.

1. How many milliliters of fluid should a 7-year-old child receive each day?

2. A child weighs 5.5 kg. How many milliliters of fluid does the child need for daily maintenance?

3. A 6-month-old girl weighs 6 kg. What is the range of fluid the girl should receive in 24 hours?

4. How many milliliters of fluid does a child with a calorie requirement of 1,200 kcal/day need?

5. How many milliliters of fluid does a child with a BSA of 0.45 m² require every day?

6. What is the minimum volume of fluid a 50-lb boy should receive each day?

7. What is the minimum daily volume of fluid that an infant weighing 8 lb requires?

8. A child's calorie requirement is 700 kcal/day. What is the child's daily maintenance fluid requirement?

9. How many milliliters of fluid per day does a 14-year-old boy require?

10. How many milliliters of fluid does a child weighing 18 kg require daily?

Review problems

Answer the following questions about pediatric dosages. To check your answers, see page 236.

1. The suggested dosage of tobramycin (Nebcin) is 4 mg/kg/day for a neonate who weighs 3 kg. If the dosage must be divided and given every 12 hours, how many milligrams will the child receive in each dose?

2. A doctor prescribes 7.5 mg/kg of amikacin (Amikin) every 12 hours for a 4-kg infant. How many milligrams of the drug will the infant receive each day?

3. If the suggested dosage of chloramphenicol (Chloromycetin) is 50 mg/kg/day in divided doses every 6 hours, how many milligrams should the nurse give at each dose to a 17-kg child?

4. If the suggested dosage of thioridazine (Mellaril) is 1.5 mg/kg/day, how many milligrams would the nurse administer daily to a 16-kg child?

5. A child who is 35″ tall and weighs 60 lb is to receive prednisone (Deltasone) 60 mg/m² daily for 4 to 6 weeks until remission. What is the child's BSA? What will the dose be?

6. If the average adult dosage of cytarabine (Cytosar-U) is 350 mg daily for 5 days by continuous I.V. infusion, how many milligrams daily should a child whose BSA is 0.9 m² receive?

7. If the average adult dose of doxorubicin (Adriamycin RDF) is 100 mg I.V., how many milligrams will a child with a BSA of 0.33 m² require?

8. A full-term infant weighing 7 lb is to receive an ordered dose of 25 mcg/kg of digoxin (Lanoxin) pediatric elixir. If the usual adult oral digitalizing dose is 0.5 to 0.75 mg, verify that the ordered infant dose is within safe limits, using the BSA method. How many micrograms will the ordered dose deliver? What is the safe range for this infant?

9. If the average adult dose of kanamycin (Kantrex) injection is 500 mg, how many milligrams would the nurse give to a child age 2 years?

10. If the average adult dose of aluminum hydroxide (Amphojel) suspension is 30 ml, how many milliliters would the nurse give to a 3-year-old child?

11. If the average adult dose of acetaminophen (Tylenol) solution is 650 mg, how many milligrams should the nurse give to a 44-lb child?

12. If the average adult dose of phenobarbital (Barbita) elixir is 30 mg, how many milligrams should a child age 3 receive?

13. A pediatric patient is to receive 875 mg of oxacillin sodium (Bactocil) in 50 ml of fluid. The drug comes in a dosage strength of 100 mg/ml when reconstituted. If the facility's policy is to include the drug volume as part of total fluid volume, how many milliliters of diluent should the nurse add?

14. A child who weighs 28 kg needs to receive demeclocycline hydrochloride (Declomycin) 280 mg P.O. daily in two divided doses. How many milligrams should the patient receive with each dose? If the recommended daily dosage range is 6 to 12 mg/kg, does the prescribed dose fall within the range?

15. An antibiotic has just finished infusing through a central venous line with a volume control set. How many milliliters of fluid should the nurse use to flush the line?

16. The doctor orders carbamazepine (Tegretol) 900 mg P.O. daily in four divided doses for a pediatric patient with seizures who weighs 30 kg. How many milligrams of the drug should the patient receive with each dose? The recommended dosage range is 10 to 20 mg/kg P.O. daily. Does the prescribed dose fall within this range?

17. Miconazole (Monistat) is provided in a formulation of 10 mg/ml. The patient must receive 500 mg of this drug in 200 ml of fluid. If the drug volume is included in the diluent volume, how many milliliters of diluent should the nurse add?

18. A child has a BSA of 0.52 m². How many milliliters of fluid will meet the child's daily maintenance fluid requirements?

19. An 8-month-old boy weighs 16 lb. What is the minimum *and* maximum volume of fluid he should receive daily?

20. A child weighs 37 kg. How much fluid should the nurse provide over 24 hours to meet the child's needs?

21. A pediatric patient uses 1,300 calories per day. What are the child's daily fluid requirements?

22. A pediatric patient has a BSA of 0.8 m². How much fluid does this patient require each day?

23. How much fluid does a 2-year-old require each day?

24. For a child, age 4 months, who weighs 4.5 kg, what range of fluid volume is appropriate to administer?

25. A 60-lb child should receive how much fluid to maintain fluid balance?

Answers to practice problems

◆ Pediatric patients and drugs

1. the same
2. medication dropper
3. mixed
4. immunizations
5. 1 ml

◆ Calculating pediatric dosages

1. 30.45 or 30.5 kg
2. 4.2 kg
3. 136 mg
4. 511.5 mg
5. 135 mg
6. 1,500 mg

7. 1 tablet

8. 0.66 m²

9. 0.82 m²

10. 1.4 m²

11. 4.59 or 4.6 mg

12. 275 mg

13. 1 tablet

14. 4.5 ml

◆ *Other calculations for pediatric dosages*

1. a) 2.2 or 2 ml

b) 2.66 or 2.7 mg

2. a) 8 mg

b) 88.3 or 88 mcg

3. a) 257 mg (give 250 mg)

b) 35.9 mg (give 35 mg)

4. a) 600 mg I.V. daily; 150 mg

b) 800 mg I.V. daily; 200 mg

c) No

5. Yes. The recommended dosage range is 60 to 224 mg/day, and the recommended range per dose is 10 to 37 mg every 4 hours.

◆ *Following pediatric guidelines and protocols*

1. 15 ml; 20 ml

2. 23 ml

3. No, the recommended dose for a 35-kg child is 105 mg I.V. daily in four divided doses.

4. microdrip

5. 60 gtt/min

◆ *Calculating pediatric fluid needs*

1. 1,600 ml

2. 550 ml

3. 750 to 900 ml

4. 1,440 ml

5. 675 ml

6. 1,554 ml

7. 363.6 or 364 ml

8. 840 ml

9. 2,300 ml

10. 1,400 ml

Answers to review problems

1. 6 mg

2. 60 mg

3. 212.5 or 213 mg

4. 24 mg

5. Based on a BSA of 0.87 m², the dose should be 52.2 or 52 mg.

6. 182 mg

7. 19 mg

8. 80 mcg; safe range is 64 mcg to 95 mcg

9. 40 mg

10. 1 ml

11. 190.7 or 191 mg (give 190 mg)

12. 6 mg

13. 41.25 ml

14. 140 mg; yes, because the recommended daily dosage range is 168 to 336 mg, and the recommended range per dose is 84 to 168 mg.

15. 20 ml

16. 225 mg; no, because the recommended daily dosage range is 300 to 600 mg, and the recommended range per dose is 75 to 150 mg. The nurse should notify the doctor.

17. 150 ml

18. 780 ml

19. 913 to 1,095 ml

20. 1,840 ml

21. 1,560 ml

22. 1,200 ml

23. 1,100 ml

24. 563 to 675 ml

25. 1,640 ml

Chapter

21

◆

Dosages for Obstetric Patients

Drug administration to obstetric patients poses special challenges because the nurse must consider two patients at once — the mother and the fetus — and because this leaves a very narrow margin for error. Chapter 21 begins by reviewing drugs that are commonly used in labor and delivery. Then it demonstrates dosage calculations for these specialized drugs. Through patient situations, the chapter shows how the nurse can titrate dosages safely to prevent or induce labor.

Commonly used drugs

In labor and delivery, drugs are commonly used to reverse the effects of pregnancy-induced hypertension (PIH), inhibit preterm labor, induce labor, and prevent postpartal hemorrhage. Because any drug administered to the mother can affect the fetus, use of these drugs warrants careful monitoring of the mother and her fetus.

When monitoring the mother, the nurse should frequently check vital signs, urine output, uterine contractions, and deep tendon reflexes. Fluid monitoring is especially important because of decreased renal function in the mother with PIH and the antidiuretic effect of the drugs used to inhibit preterm labor. Assessing breath sounds and monitoring fluid intake and output can help reduce the mother's risk of fluid overload, which may lead to acute pulmonary edema.

To evaluate the fetus's response to treatment, the nurse should continuously monitor fetal heart tones. A sudden increase or decrease in fetal heart rate may signify an adverse reaction to treatment, requiring immediate drug discontinuation.

Drugs used to inhibit preterm labor include ritodrine hydrochloride (Yutopar) and terbutaline sulfate (Brethine). They stimulate the beta$_2$-adrenergic receptors in uterine smooth muscle, thereby inhibiting contractility. To administer one of these drugs, mix it in a compatible intravenous (I.V.) solution and administer it via infusion pump. Then titrate the dose every 10 minutes until the contractions subside or the maximum dose is reached.

Magnesium sulfate is used to prevent or control seizures caused by PIH. The drug may act by decreasing acetylcholine levels, but its exact anticonvulsant mechanism is unknown. To administer magnesium sulfate, first give a loading dose (a high dose administered over a short time) to reach a therapeutic drug level. Then, give a maintenance infusion at a lower dose, as prescribed. During the infusion, closely assess knee jerk and patellar reflexes; loss of these reflexes signifies drug toxicity. If toxicity occurs, expect to administer calcium gluconate (Kalcinate) as an antidote.

The most commonly used drug to induce labor, oxytocin (Pitocin) works by selectively stimulating uterine smooth muscle. After mixing it with a compatible solution, administer oxytocin by I.V. infusion pump and titrate it until a normal contraction pattern occurs. When labor is firmly established, decrease the infusion rate. During the infusion, carefully monitor contraction strength because the drug can cause severe contractions that may lead to uterine rupture — and fetal and maternal death.

After delivery of the placenta, oxytocin may be used to control bleeding. To accomplish this, add the drug to 1 L of I.V. fluid or as prescribed. Then infuse it at a rate that controls bleeding, but does not exceed 20 mU/min.

◆ PRACTICE PROBLEMS

Commonly used drugs

Fill in the blanks in the following statements about commonly used drugs in labor and delivery. To check your answers, see page 242.

1. For a patient in preterm labor, the doctor prescribes an infusion of ritodrine hydrochloride (Yutopar). The nurse should administer this drug via

   _____ _____ .

2. While monitoring a patient who is receiving ritodrine HCL to inhibit preterm labor, the nurse should assess for signs of fluid overload, which may lead to _____ edema.

3. Before receiving a maintenance infusion of magnesium sulfate, the patient should receive a _____ _____ .

4. Drugs administered to a patient during labor can affect her and the

   _____ .

5. The antidote for magnesium sulfate toxicity is _____ .

Calculating dosages

In the labor and delivery unit, the nurse must be especially careful to calculate and administer medications accurately for two main reasons. First, the obstetric nurse may be dealing with life-threatening problems, such as hemorrhage or seizures caused by PIH. Because of this similarity to critical care, the nurse uses the same methods for calculating dosages in labor and delivery as in critical care. Second, the nurse is caring for two patients at once — the mother and the fetus. By administering accurate dosages to the mother, the nurse helps avoid fetal complications.

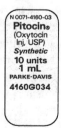

Patient situations

A doctor prescribes oxytocin, as follows, to stimulate labor: 1 ml (10 U) oxytocin (Pitocin) in 1 L NSS; infuse at 2 mU/min for 20 minutes, then increase flow rate to 3 mU/min. The nurse must give Pitocin, as shown on the label above, via an infusion pump. What is the solution's concentration? What is the flow rate needed to deliver 2 mU/min for 20 minutes? What is the flow rate needed to deliver 3 mU/min thereafter?

◆ Determine the solution's concentration by using the following proportion and solving for X.

$$\frac{10\ U}{1,000\ ml} = \frac{X\ U}{1\ ml}$$

$$X\ U \times 1,000\ ml = 10\ U \times 1\ ml$$

$$X = \frac{10\ U}{1,000}$$

$$X = 0.01\ U$$

This can be written in milliunits (mU, thousandths of a unit). In this case, 0.01 U = 10 mU, so the concentration is 10 mU/ml.

◆ If the patient is to receive 2 mU/min for 20 minutes, a total of 40 mU should be received. To calculate the flow rate needed to provide that dose, use the following proportion and solve for X.

$$\frac{10\ mU}{1\ ml} = \frac{40\ mU}{X\ ml}$$

$$X\ ml \times 10\ mU = 1\ ml \times 40\ mU$$

$$X = \frac{40\ ml}{10}$$

$$X = 4\ ml$$

The flow rate should be 4 ml/20 min. Because an infusion pump must be used to deliver this medication, compute the hourly flow rate.

◆ Multiply the 20-minute rate by 3.

$$4\ ml/20\ min \times 3 = 12\ ml/hr$$

◆ Remember to change this rate after 20 minutes. Calculate the flow rate to be used after the first 20 minutes to provide 3 mU/min (or 180 mU/hr). Having calculated the solution's concentration as 10 mU/ml, use the following proportion and solve for X.

$$\frac{10\ mU}{1\ ml} = \frac{180\ mU}{X\ ml}$$

$$X\ ml \times 10\ mU = 1\ ml \times 180\ mU$$

$$X = \frac{180\ ml}{10}$$

$$X = 18\ ml$$

After 20 minutes, reset the pump to deliver 18 ml/hr.

A doctor orders magnesium sulfate, 4 g in 250 ml D₅W, to be infused at 2 g/hour. What is the flow rate (in ml/hr)?

◆ One approach is to use the following proportion and solve for X.

$$\frac{4\ g}{250\ ml} = \frac{2\ g}{X\ ml}$$

$$X\ ml \times 4\ g = 250\ ml \times 2\ g$$

$$X = \frac{500\ ml}{4}$$

$$X = 125\ ml$$

The magnesium sulfate solution should be infused at 125 ml/hr.

◆ Another approach is to calculate the strength of the solution.

$$\frac{4 \text{ g}}{250 \text{ ml}} = \frac{X \text{ g}}{1 \text{ ml}}$$

$$X \text{ ml} \times 250 \text{ ml} = 4 \text{ g} \times 1 \text{ ml}$$

$$X = \frac{4 \text{ g}}{250}$$

$$X = 0.016 \text{ g}$$

◆ Next, calculate the flow rate as follows and solve for X.

$$\frac{X \text{ ml}}{2 \text{ g}} = \frac{1 \text{ ml}}{0.016 \text{ g}}$$

$$X \text{ ml} \times 0.016 \text{ g} = 1 \text{ ml} \times 2 \text{ g}$$

$$X = \frac{2 \text{ ml}}{0.016}$$

$$X = 125 \text{ ml}$$

Note that the same flow rate (125 ml/hour) is obtained using either method.

For a patient with preterm labor, the doctor prescribes ritodrine hydrochloride (Yutopar) 150 mg in 500 ml of D_5W I.V. to infuse at 0.35 mg/min. What flow rate should the nurse use to administer this dose?

◆ To find the solution's strength, use the following proportion and solve for X.

$$\frac{X \text{ mg}}{1 \text{ ml}} = \frac{150 \text{ mg}}{400 \text{ ml}}$$

$$X \text{ mg} \times 500 \text{ ml} = 1 \text{ ml} \times 150 \text{ mg}$$

$$X = \frac{150 \text{ mg}}{500}$$

$$X = 0.3 \text{ mg}$$

The solution's strength is 0.3 mg/ml.

◆ Next, calculate the flow rate needed to deliver the prescribed dose of 0.35 mg/min. To do this, use the following proportion and solve for X.

$$\frac{X \text{ ml}}{0.35 \text{ mg}} = \frac{1 \text{ ml}}{0.3 \text{ mg}}$$

$$X \text{ ml} \times 0.3 \text{ mg} = 0.35 \text{ mg} \times 1 \text{ ml}$$

$$X = \frac{0.35 \text{ ml}}{0.3}$$

$$X = 1.16 \text{ ml, rounded to 1 ml}$$

The flow rate is 1 ml/min.

◆ Because an infusion pump must be used to administer ritodrine, compute the hourly flow rate.

$$\frac{X \text{ ml}}{60 \text{ min}} = \frac{1 \text{ ml}}{1 \text{ min}}$$

$$X \text{ ml} \times 1 \text{ min} = 60 \text{ min} \times 1 \text{ ml}$$

$$X = \frac{60 \text{ ml}}{1}$$

$$X = 60 \text{ ml}$$

Set the infusion pump to deliver 60 ml/hr.

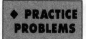

Calculating dosages

Perform the following calculations for obstetric patients. To check your answers, see page 242.

1. The doctor prescribes 1 ml (10 U) of oxytocin (Pitocin) in 1,000 ml of normal saline I.V. to infuse at 4 mU/min. What is the solution's concentration? What hourly flow rate should the nurse use to administer 4 mU/min?

2. The doctor's order states *magnesium sulfate 20 g in 1,000 ml of D_5W I.V. Infuse a loading dose of 3 g over 20 minutes followed by a maintenance infusion of 1 g/hr.* What flow rate should the nurse set on the infusion pump for the loading dose? For the maintenance dose?

3. A patient must receive terbutaline sulfate (Brethine), 10 mg in 1,000 ml of D_5W to infuse at 25 mcg/min. What hourly flow rate should the nurse use to administer the prescribed dose?

4. A patient in preterm labor is to receive 150 mg of ritodrine hydrochloride (Yutopar) in 500 ml of D_5W I.V. to infuse at 250 mcg/min. What is the solution's concentration? What rate should the nurse set on the infusion pump to deliver this dose?

Review problems

Answer the following questions about dosages in obstetric patients. To check your answers, see page 242.

1. Patients with PIH have decreased _____ function.

2. A sudden change in fetal heart rate may signify an adverse reaction to a drug, requiring its immediate _____ .

3. Drugs used to _____ preterm labor include ritodrine hydrochloride (Yutopar) and terbutaline sulfate (Brethine).

4. The nurse should keep calcium gluconate handy when administering _____ to an obstetric patient.

5. The doctor's order states *10 U Pitocin in 1,000 ml NS; infuse at 4 mU/min.* What is the solution's concentration (in mU/ml)? What should the infusion rate be per minute? Per hour?

6. The doctor orders 500 mg/hr of magnesium sulfate. The 500-ml I.V. bag contains 4 g of the drug. What is the solution's concentration (in mg/ml)? What is the hourly infusion rate?

7. A patient is to receive oxytocin as follows: 4 mU/min for 20 minutes, followed by 6 NSS mU/min for 20 minutes. The label on the 500-ml bag of normal saline reads *oxytocin 10 units.* What is the solution's concentration (in mU/ml)? What flow rate should the infusion pump be set to deliver for the first 20 minutes? For the next 20 minutes?

8. The patient in preterm labor must receive 150 mg of ritrodrine hydrochloride (Yutopar) in 500 ml of D_5W, beginning with an infusion of 100 mcg/min and increasing by 50 mcg/min every 10 minutes until contractions cease or a maximum of 350 mcg/min is provided. What is the hourly flow rate of the starting dose? What is the flow rate of the maximum dosage?

9. A solution contains 150 mg of ritodrine hydrochloride (Yutopar) in 1,000 ml of D_5W. What is the solution's concentration in mcg/ml?

10. The doctor's order states *Infuse terbutaline sulfate 10 mg in 1,000 ml of D_5W at 0.01 mg/ min for 20 minutes, then increase to 0.02 mg/min.* What is the flow rate (in ml/hr) for the first 20 minutes? What is the flow rate after that?

11. A solution contains 40 U of oxytocin (Pitocin) in 1,000 ml of D_5W. What is the solution's concentration in mU/ml?

Answers to practice problems

◆ Commonly used drugs
1. infusion pump
2. pulmonary
3. loading dose
4. fetus
5. calcium gluconate (Kalcinate)

◆ Calculating dosages
1. 0.01 U/ml or 10 mU/ml; 24 ml/hr
2. 450 ml/hr; 50 ml/hr
3. 150 ml/hr
4. 0.3 mg/ml or 300 mcg/ml; 50 ml/hr

Answers to review problems

1. renal
2. discontinuation
3. inhibit
4. magnesium sulfate
5. 10 mU/ml; 0.4 ml/min; 24 ml/hr
6. 8 mg/ml; 63 ml/hr
7. 20 mU/ml; 12 ml/hr for the first 20 minutes; 18 ml/hr for the next 20 minutes
8. 18 ml/hr; 72 ml/hr
9. 150 mcg/ml
10. 60 ml/hr; 120 ml/hr
11. 40 mU/ml

Chapter

22

◆

Dosages for Critical Care Patients

Many drugs are administered by the intravenous (I.V.) route to critical care patients in life-threatening situations. Therefore, the nurse in a critical care unit must be able to perform dosage calculations quickly and accurately. Chapter 22 will help prepare the nurse for these responsibilities by presenting calculations for I.V. push drugs and I.V. flow rates for specialized drugs.

Calculating dosages for I.V. push drugs

In critical care units, the nurse commonly administers drugs to rapidly control heart rate, respirations, blood pressure, cardiac output, or kidney function. These potent, fast-acting drugs generally have a short duration of action, which enables the nurse to evaluate their effectiveness immediately and, if they are ineffective, begin other treatments.

Dosage calculations for I.V. push drugs used in critical care are the same as calculations for other I.V. push drugs. However, the nurse must perform calculation with extra care because of the potency and potential adverse effects of these drugs. Also, the nurse must check for special instructions related to administration of the specific drug *before* administering it.

Patient situations

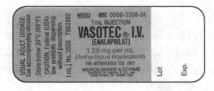

For a hypertensive patient, the doctor orders enalaprilat (Vasotec I.V.) 2.5 mg I.V. STAT. This drug is contained in packages like the one pictured above. How many milliliters of the drug should the nurse administer?

♦ Using fractions, set up the proportion.

$$\frac{2.5 \text{ mg}}{X \text{ ml}} = \frac{1.25 \text{ g}}{1 \text{ ml}}$$

◆ Solve for X.

$$X \text{ ml} \times 1.25 \text{ mg} = 2.5 \text{ mg} \times 1 \text{ ml}$$

$$X = \frac{2.5 \text{ ml}}{1.25}$$

$$X = 2 \text{ ml}$$

The nurse should administer 2 ml or 2 vials of the solution. According to the special administration instructions, the nurse must give the drug slowly, administering each 1.25 mg of the drug over 5 minutes.

After undergoing a thoracotomy, a patient suddenly develops supraventricular tachycardia, as shown on his electrocardiogram (ECG) tracing. The doctor orders verapamil hydrochloride (Isoptin) 5 mg I.V. push STAT. The pharmacy dispenses the drug in a dosage strength of 2.5 mg/ml. How many milliliters of the drug should the patient receive?

◆ Using fractions, set up the proportion.

$$\frac{5 \text{ mg}}{X \text{ ml}} = \frac{2.5 \text{ mg}}{1 \text{ ml}}$$

◆ Solve for X.

$$X \text{ ml} \times 2.5 \text{ mg} = 5 \text{ mg} \times 1 \text{ ml}$$

$$X = \frac{5 \text{ ml}}{2.5}$$

$$X = 2 \text{ ml}$$

The patient should receive 2 ml of the verapamil hydrochloride solution.

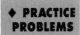 **◆ PRACTICE PROBLEMS**

Calculating dosages for I.V. push drugs

Perform the following dosage calculations related to I.V. push drugs. To check your answers, see page 253.

1. The doctor prescribes midazolam hydrochloride (Versed) 2 mg I.V. STAT for a severely agitated patient on mechanical ventilation. The drug is available in a dosage strength of 5 mg/ml. How many milliliters of the drug should the nurse administer?

2. For a patient with symptomatic bradycardia, the nurse must administer atropine sulfate 0.5 mg I.V. The available dosage strength is 1 mg/ml. How many milliliters should the nurse administer?

3. When a patient is admitted with a myocardial infarction, the doctor orders metoprolol tartrate (Lopressor) 5 mg I.V. The pharmacist dispenses the drug in a 5-ml ampule with a dosage strength of 1 mg/ml. How many milliliters of the drug should the patient receive?

4. A patient with severe hypertension needs to receive hydralazine hydrochloride (Apresoline) 15 mg I.V. STAT. The drug is supplied in a dosage strength of 20 mg/ml. How many milliliters of the drug should the patient receive?

5. For an intubated patient with increased intracranial pressure, the doctor orders pentobarbital (Nembutal) 100 mg I.V. every hour. The drug's dosage strength is 50 mg/ml. How many milliliters of the drug should the patient receive with each dose?

Calculating I.V. flow rates

In the critical care unit, the nurse must perform calculations for medication additives quickly. Many I.V. drugs—such as the antiarrhythmics lidocaine and bretylium, the vasodilators sodium nitroprusside and nitroglycerin, and the adrenergics norepinephrine and dopamine—are administered in life-threatening situations. The nurse must prepare the drug for infusion, administer it to the patient, and observe the patient to evaluate the drug's effectiveness.

For example, one or more adrenergic drugs usually are given to a patient in shock to raise cardiac output quickly. Adrenergic medications, given in 250, 500, or 1,000 ml of I.V. solution, typically are ordered in micrograms per minute or micrograms per kilogram per minute. They must be given via infusion pumps, and the flow rate must be adjusted, or titrated, to restore and maintain normal blood pressure. If more than one adrenergic drug is ordered, each must be diluted and infused in a separate solution.

When administering these types of medications, the nurse must calculate the drug's concentration in the I.V. solution and the flow rate required to deliver the desired dose. The nurse also may have to calculate the number of micrograms needed, based on the patient's weight in kilograms.

To calculate the drug's concentration, use the following equation.

$$\text{concentration (in mg/ml)} = \frac{\text{mg of medication}}{\text{ml of fluid}}$$

To convert the concentration from milligrams to micrograms, multiply by 1,000.

The nurse can use either of two methods to calculate the I.V. flow rate. In one method, determine the flow rate per minute, using the following proportion.

$$\frac{\text{dose/minute}}{\text{X ml/min}} = \frac{\text{concentration of solution}}{\text{1 ml of fluid}}$$

In the other method, first multiply the ordered dose, given in micrograms per minute, by 60 minutes to determine the hourly dose. Next, use the following proportion to compute the hourly flow rate.

$$\frac{\text{hourly dose}}{\text{X ml/hr}} = \frac{\text{concentration of solution}}{\text{1 ml of fluid}}$$

To ensure that the drug is being given within a safe and therapeutic range, determine the amount of medication given (in mg/kg/min) and compare it to information shown in a drug reference. That calculation involves several steps.

♦ First, determine the solution's concentration, as explained above. Then, determine the amount of medication being given to the patient by multiplying the flow rate by the concentration.

$$\text{medication received (mg/hr)} = \text{flow rate} \times \text{concentration}$$

♦ Next, calculate the dose being received by the patient each minute. To do this, divide the hourly amount by 60 minutes.

$$\text{mg/min} = \frac{\text{mg/hr}}{\text{60 min}}$$

♦ Then, divide the amount of medication delivered each minute by the patient's weight.

$$\text{mg/kg/min} = \frac{\text{mg/min}}{\text{weight (kg)}}$$

Compare this amount to the dosage information in a drug reference.

Patient situations

A doctor's order for a patient with cardiac arrhythmias states **Administer lidocaine hydrochloride (Xylocaine) 2 g in 500 ml of D$_5$W to infuse at 2 mg/min.** *What is the flow rate in milliliters per minute? In milliliters per hour?*

◆ To find the solution's concentration, use the following proportion and solve for X.

$$\frac{X \text{ mg}}{1 \text{ ml}} = \frac{2{,}000 \text{ mg}}{500 \text{ ml}}$$

$$X \text{ mg} \times 500 \text{ ml} = 1 \text{ ml} \times 2{,}000 \text{ mg}$$

$$X = \frac{2{,}000 \text{ mg}}{500}$$

$$X = 4 \text{ mg}$$

The solution's concentration is 4 mg/ml.

◆ To calculate the flow rate (per minute) needed to deliver the ordered dose of 2 mg/min, use the following proportion and solve for X.

$$\frac{2 \text{ mg}}{X \text{ ml}} = \frac{4 \text{ mg}}{1 \text{ ml}}$$

$$X \text{ ml} \times 4 \text{ mg} = 2 \text{ mg} \times 1 \text{ ml}$$

$$X = \frac{2 \text{ ml}}{4}$$

$$X = 0.5 \text{ ml}$$

The patient should receive 0.5 ml/min.

◆ Because an infusion pump must be used when administering lidocaine, compute the hourly flow rate by using the following proportion and solving for X.

$$\frac{X \text{ ml}}{60 \text{ min}} = \frac{0.5 \text{ ml}}{1 \text{ min}}$$

◆ Solve for X.

$$X \text{ ml} \times 1 \text{ min} = 60 \text{ min} \times 0.5 \text{ ml}$$

$$X = \frac{60 \text{ min} \times 0.5 \text{ ml}}{1 \text{ min}}$$

$$X = \frac{30 \text{ ml}}{1}$$

$$X = 30 \text{ ml}$$

Set the infusion pump to deliver 30 ml/hr.

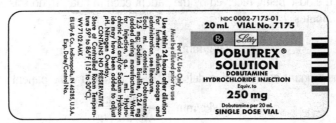

A 200-lb patient must receive an I.V. infusion of dobutamine (Dobutrex) at 10 mcg/kg/min. Based on the doctor's order and the drug label (see above), the nurse dilutes 250 mg of dobutamine in 50 ml of D$_5$W. Because the drug vial contains 20 ml of solu-

tion, the total volume to be infused is 70 ml. How many milligrams of the drug should the patient receive each minute? Each hour? What should the hourly flow rate be?

◆ Determine the amount of dobutamine the patient should receive each minute. First, compute the patient's weight in kilograms.

$$\frac{200 \text{ lb}}{X \text{ kg}} = \frac{2.2 \text{ lb}}{1 \text{ kg}}$$

◆ Solve for X.

$$X \text{ kg} \times 2.2 \text{ lb} = 200 \text{ lb} \times 1 \text{ kg}$$

$$X = \frac{200 \text{ lb} \times 1 \text{ kg}}{2.2 \text{ lb}}$$

$$X = \frac{200 \text{ kg}}{2.2}$$

$$X = 90.9 \text{ kg}$$

◆ Because the patient needs to receive 10 mcg/kg/min, use the following proportion and solve for X to determine the dose per minute.

$$\frac{90.9 \text{ kg}}{X \text{ mcg}} = \frac{1 \text{ kg}}{10 \text{ mcg}}$$

$$X \text{ mcg} \times 1 \text{ kg} = 90.9 \text{ kg} \times 10 \text{ mcg}$$

$$X = \frac{90.9 \text{ kg} \times 10 \text{ mcg}}{1 \text{ kg}}$$

$$X = 909 \text{ mcg}$$

The patient should receive 909 mcg/min or 0.909 mg/min.

◆ To determine the hourly dose, multiply the dose/minute by 60.

$$909 \text{ mcg/min} \times 60 \text{ min/hr} = 54,540 \text{ mcg/hr}$$

The patient should receive 54,540 mcg, or 54.54 mg of dobutamine every hour.

◆ To find the solution's concentration, use the following proportion and solve for X.

$$\frac{X \text{ mg}}{1 \text{ ml}} = \frac{250 \text{ mg}}{70 \text{ ml}}$$

$$X \text{ mg} \times 70 \text{ ml} = 1 \text{ ml} \times 250 \text{ mg}$$

$$X = \frac{1 \text{ ml} \times 250 \text{ mg}}{70 \text{ ml}}$$

$$X = \frac{250 \text{ mg}}{70}$$

$$X = 3.57, \text{ or } 3.6 \text{ mg}$$

The concentration of the solution is 3.6 mg/ml.

◆ To calculate the flow rate needed to deliver the ordered dose of 54.54 mg/hr, use the following proportion and solve for X.

$$\frac{54.54 \text{ mg}}{X \text{ ml}} = \frac{3.6 \text{ mg}}{1 \text{ ml}}$$

$$X \text{ ml} \times 3.6 \text{ mg} = 54.54 \text{ mg} \times 1 \text{ ml}$$

$$X = \frac{54.54 \text{ mg} \times 1 \text{ ml}}{3.6 \text{ mg}}$$

$$X = \frac{54.54 \text{ mg}}{3.6}$$

$$X = 15.15, \text{ or } 15 \text{ ml}$$

The patient should receive 15 ml/hr.

A doctor's order for a 200-lb patient states sodium nitroprusside (Nipride); dilute **50 mg in 250 ml D₅W and administer at 3 mcg/kg/min.** *What is the infusion rate in milliliters per hour?*

◆ Convert the patient's weight in pounds to kilograms.

$$200 \text{ lb} \div 2.2 \text{ kg/lb} = 90.9 \text{ kg}$$

◆ Because the patient is to receive 3 mcg/kg/min, use the following proportion to determine the dose per minute.

$$\frac{90.9 \text{ kg}}{X \text{ mcg/min}} = \frac{1 \text{ kg}}{3 \text{ mcg/min}}$$

$$X \text{ mcg/min} \times 1 \text{ kg} = 90.9 \text{ kg} \times 3 \text{ mcg/min}$$

$$X = 27, 2.7, \text{ or } 273 \text{ mcg/min}$$

◆ To determine the hourly dose, multiply the dose/minute by 60.

$$273 \text{ mcg/min} \times 60 \text{ min/hr} = 16,380 \text{ mcg/hr}$$

◆ To find the solution's concentration, use the following proportion and solve for X.

$$\frac{X \text{ mg}}{1 \text{ ml}} = \frac{50 \text{ mg}}{250 \text{ ml}}$$

$$X \text{ mg} \times 250 \text{ ml} = 1 \text{ ml} \times 50 \text{ mg}$$

$$X = \frac{50 \text{ mg}}{250 \text{ ml}}$$

$$X = 0.2 \text{ mg/ml}$$

The solution contains 0.2 mg/ml, or 200 mcg/ml.

◆ To calculate the flow rate needed to deliver the ordered dose of 16,380 mcg/hr, use the following proportion and solve for X.

$$\frac{16,380 \text{ mcg}}{X \text{ ml}} = \frac{200 \text{ mcg}}{1 \text{ ml}}$$

$$X \text{ ml} \times 200 \text{ mcg} = 16,380 \text{ mcg} \times 1 \text{ ml}$$

$$X = \frac{16,380 \text{ ml}}{200}$$

$$X = 81.9, \text{ or } 82 \text{ ml/hr}$$

A doctor's order for a patient states Administer 125 mg nitroglycerin (Nitrostat) in 500 ml **D₅W. Administer at 10 ml/hr.** *Check to ensure that this hourly flow rate will deliver approximately 42 mcg/min.*

◆ Multiply the safe dose (stated on the drug label or package information) by 60 to determine the safe hourly dose.

$$42 \text{ mcg/min} \times 60 \text{ min/hr} = 2,520 \text{ mcg/hr}$$

♦ To find the solution's strength, use the following proportion and solve for X.

$$\frac{X \text{ mg}}{1 \text{ ml}} = \frac{125 \text{ mg}}{500 \text{ ml}}$$

$$X \text{ mg} \times 500 \text{ ml} = 1 \text{ ml} \times 125 \text{ mg}$$

$$X = \frac{125 \text{ mg}}{500 \text{ ml}}$$

$$X = 0.25 \text{ mg/ml}$$

♦ To determine the hourly dose being received at the ordered flow rate, use the following proportion and solve for X.

$$\frac{10 \text{ ml}}{X \text{ mcg}} = \frac{1 \text{ ml}}{250 \text{ mcg}}$$

$$X \text{ mcg} \times 1 \text{ ml} = 10 \text{ ml} \times 250 \text{ mcg}$$

$$X = 2,500 \text{ mcg}$$

The patient is receiving 2,500 mcg/hr. This is approximately equal to the desired dosage of 2,520 mcg (stated on the drug label or package information).

A doctor's order for a 200-lb (90.9 kg) patient states* Administer 1 amp (200 mg) dopamine (Intropin) in 250 ml D₅W. Administer at 34 ml/hr. *The hourly flow rate should deliver approximately 5 mcg/kg/min.

♦ Multiply the safe dose by the patient's weight in kilograms to determine the dose per minute.

$$90.9 \text{ kg} \times 5 \text{ mcg/kg/min} = 454.5 \text{ mcg/min}$$

♦ Multiply this dose by 60 to determine the safe hourly dose.

$$454.5 \text{ mcg/min} \times 60 \text{ min/hr} = 27,270 \text{ mcg/hr}$$

♦ To find the solution's concentration, use the following proportion and solve for X.

$$\frac{X \text{ mg}}{1 \text{ ml}} = \frac{200 \text{ mg}}{250 \text{ ml}}$$

$$X \text{ mg} \times 250 \text{ ml} = 1 \text{ ml} \times 200 \text{ mg}$$

$$X = \frac{200 \text{ mg}}{250 \text{ ml}}$$

$$X = 0.8 \text{ mg/ml or } 800 \text{ mcg/ml}$$

The solution contains 0.8 mg, or 800 mcg of dopamine per milliliter.

♦ To determine the hourly dose being received at the ordered flow rate, use the following proportion and solve for X.

$$\frac{34 \text{ ml}}{X \text{ mcg}} = \frac{1 \text{ ml}}{800 \text{ mcg}}$$

$$X \text{ mcg} \times 1 \text{ ml} = 34 \text{ ml} \times 800 \text{ mcg}$$

$$X = 27,200 \text{ mcg}$$

The nurse is caring for a patient who is receiving diltiazem hydrochloride (Cardizem) I.V. at 10 ml/hr. The solution contains 100 mg of the drug in 100 ml of D₅W. How many milligrams per hour is the patient receiving?

♦ To find the solution's concentration, use the following proportion and solve for X.

$$\frac{X \text{ mg}}{1 \text{ ml}} = \frac{100 \text{ mg}}{100 \text{ ml}}$$

$$X \text{ mg} \times 1 \text{ ml} = 1 \text{ ml} \times 100 \text{ mg}$$

$$X = \frac{100 \text{ mg}}{100 \text{ ml}}$$

$$X = 1 \text{ mg/ml}$$

♦ To determine the hourly dose being delivered at a flow rate of 10 ml/hr, use the following proportion and solve for X.

$$\frac{10 \text{ ml}}{X \text{ mg}} = \frac{1 \text{ ml}}{1 \text{ mg}}$$

$$X \text{ mg} \times 1 \text{ ml} = 10 \text{ ml} \times 1 \text{ mg}$$

$$X = 10 \text{ mg}$$

The patient is receiving 10 mg/hr when the flow rate is set at 10 ml/hr.

Special considerations

Sometimes, critical care drugs are not ordered at a specific flow rate or dosage. Instead, they are prescribed based on specific parameters, such as heart rate or blood pressure. When this must be done, the doctor orders a starting dose and a maximum dose to which the drug can be titrated. For example, a doctor's order may state *dopamine hydrochloride (Dopastat) 800 mg in 500 ml of D_5W, start at 3 mcg/kg/min titrate to maintain systolic blood pressure > 90 mm Hg. May titrate to a maximum of 10 mcg/kg/min.* To deliver the correct amount of medication, the nurse must calculate the starting dose and the maximum dose.

Patient situation

For a patient who weighs 85 kg, the doctor prescribes **nitroprusside sodium (Nipride) 50 mg in 250 ml of D_5W. Start at 0.5 mcg/kg/min. Titrate to keep systolic BP < 170 mm Hg. Maximum dose is 5 mcg/kg/min.**

♦ Because the starting dose is 0.5 mcg/kg/min, use the following proportion and solve for X to determine the dose per minute.

$$\frac{85 \text{ kg}}{X \text{ mcg}} = \frac{1 \text{ kg}}{0.5 \text{ mcg}}$$

$$X \text{ mcg} \times 1 \text{ kg} = 85 \text{ kg} \times 0.5 \text{ mcg}$$

$$X = \frac{85 \text{ kg} \times 0.5 \text{ mcg}}{1 \text{ kg}}$$

$$X = 42.5 \text{ mcg}$$

The starting dose is 42.5 mcg/min.

♦ To determine the hourly starting dose, multiply the dose per minute by 60.

$$42.5 \text{ mcg/min} \times 60 \text{ min/hr} = 2,550 \text{ mcg/hr, or } 2.55 \text{ mg/hr}$$

♦ To find the solution's concentration, use the following proportion and solve for X.

$$\frac{X \text{ mg}}{1 \text{ ml}} = \frac{50 \text{ mg}}{250 \text{ ml}}$$

$$X \text{ mg} \times 250 \text{ ml} = 1 \text{ ml} \times 50 \text{ mg}$$

$$X = \frac{1 \text{ ml} \times 50 \text{ mg}}{250 \text{ ml}}$$

$$X = 0.2 \text{ mg, or } 200 \text{ mcg}$$

The solution's concentration is 200 mcg/ml.

◆ To calculate the flow rate needed to deliver the ordered dose of 2,550 mcg/hr, use the following proportion and solve for X.

$$\frac{2,550 \text{ mcg}}{X \text{ ml}} = \frac{200 \text{ mcg}}{1 \text{ ml}}$$

$$X \text{ ml} \times 200 \text{ mcg} = 2,550 \text{ mcg} \times 1 \text{ ml}$$

$$X = \frac{2,550 \text{ mcg} \times 1 \text{ ml}}{200 \text{ mcg}}$$

$$X = 12.75 \text{ or } 13 \text{ ml}$$

The infusion should begin at a flow rate of 13 ml/hr.

◆ Next, calculate the flow rate (per minute) for the maximum dose of 5 mcg/kg/min.

$$\frac{85 \text{ kg}}{X \text{ mcg}} = \frac{1 \text{ kg}}{5 \text{ mcg}}$$

$$X \text{ mcg} \times 1 \text{ kg} = 85 \text{ kg} \times 5 \text{ mcg}$$

$$X = \frac{85 \text{ kg} \times 5 \text{ mcg}}{1 \text{ kg}}$$

$$X = 425 \text{ mcg}$$

The flow rate is 425 mcg/min.

◆ Then calculate the number of milliliters per minute to be delivered, using the following proportion and solving for X. (Remember that the solution concentration is 200 mcg/ml.)

$$\frac{200 \text{ mcg}}{1 \text{ ml}} = \frac{425 \text{ mcg}}{X \text{ ml}}$$

$$200 \text{ mcg} \times X \text{ ml} = 1 \text{ ml} \times 425 \text{ mcg}$$

$$X = \frac{1 \text{ ml} \times 425 \text{ mcg}}{200 \text{ mcg}}$$

$$X = 2.12 \text{ ml}$$

The infusion should deliver 2.12 ml/min.

◆ Now multiply the milliliters per minute by 60 to obtain the maximum hourly rate.

$$2.12 \text{ ml/min} \times 60 \text{ min/hr} = 127.2, \text{ or } 127 \text{ ml/hr}$$

The drug can be titrated to a maximum of 127 ml/hr to achieve a dose of 5 mcg/kg/hr.

Calculating I.V. flow rates

Perform the following dosage calculations related to I.V. flow rates. To check your answers, see page 253.

1. A 75-kg patient has acute renal failure and must receive dopamine hydrochloride (Dopastat) at 3 mcg/kg/min. The I.V. solution contains 800 mg of dopamine in 500 ml of D_5W. To deliver the prescribed dose, the nurse should set the infusion pump at what hourly flow rate?

2. A patient is receiving nitroglycerin (Nitrostat I.V.) I.V., titrated to 30 ml/hr to relieve pain caused by acute angina pectoris. The I.V. solution contains 200 mg of nitroglycerin in 500 ml of D_5W. How many micrograms per minute is the patient receiving?

3. A patient with septic shock is severely hypotensive. The doctor orders norepinephrine bitartrate (Levophed) 4 mg I.V. in 500 ml of D_5W at 10 mcg/min. To administer this dose, what hourly infusion rate should the nurse use?

4. For a patient with ventricular ectopy, the doctor orders lidocaine hydrochloride (Xylocaine) 2 g in 500 ml of D_5W to infuse at 15 ml/hr. How many milligrams per minute should the patient receive?

5. A patient who weighs 95 kg is admitted for treatment of severe hypertension. The doctor orders sodium nitroprusside (Nipride) 100 mg I.V. in 250 ml of D_5W, starting at 1 mcg/kg/min and being titrated to a maximum of 5 mcg/kg/min. What is the hourly flow rate at the starting dose? At the maximum dose?

Review problems

Perform the following dosage calculations used in the critical care units. To check your answers, see page 254.

1. A patient's cardiac monitor reveals paroxysmal supraventricular tachycardia. The doctor orders adenosine (Adenocard) 6 mg I.V. STAT. How many milliliters of the drug should the nurse administer if the vial contains 3 mg/ml?

2. The doctor orders metoprolol tartrate (Lopressor) 2.5 mg I.V. STAT for a patient with newly diagnosed myocardial infarction. The drug ampule contains 1 mg/ml. How many milliliters of the drug must the nurse administer to provide the ordered dose?

3. For a patient with a closed head injury, the doctor orders a loading dose of phenytoin (Dilantin) 1 g I.V. The pharmacy dispenses the drug in a dosage strength of 50 mg/ml. How many milliliters should the nurse administer?

4. For a patient with fluid overload, the doctor orders furosemide (Lasix) 80 mg I.V. The nurse has a vial with a dosage strength of 10 mg/ml. How many milliliters of the drug must the nurse administer?

5. When a patient's ECG shows uncontrolled atrial fibrillation, the doctor orders procainamide hydrochloride (Pronestyl) 2 g I.V. in 500 ml of D_5W at 3 mg/min. To administer this dose, what hourly flow rate should the nurse use?

6. To increase a patient's cardiac output, the doctor prescribes dobutamine hydrochloride (Dobutrex) 1 g I.V. in 250 ml of D_5W at 46 ml/hr. The patient weighs 60 kg. How many mcg/kg/min of the drug should the patient receive?

7. A patient is to receive a loading dose of digoxin (Lanoxin) 0.5 mg I.V., followed by 0.25 mg I.V. every 8 hours for two doses. How many milligrams should the patient receive in total?

8. A 185-lb patient with acute renal failure is receiving 800 mg of dopamine (Dobutrex) in 500 ml of D_5W at 3 mcg/kg/min. As the patient's blood pressure deteriorates, the nurse titrates the drug to 12 mcg/kg/min, as prescribed. What is the hourly flow rate initially? What is the hourly flow rate after titration?

9. The doctor's order states *lidocaine (Xylocaine) 4 g in 500 ml of D_5W to infuse at 15 ml/hr.* How many milligrams per minute should the nurse administer?

10. A patient with severe hypertension must receive 200 mg of labetalol hydrochloride (Trandate) in 200 ml of D$_5$W at 125 ml/hr. How many milligrams per minute should the patient receive?

11. The doctor's order states *nitroglycerin (Nitro-Bid I.V.) 100 mg in 500 ml of D$_5$W to infuse at 15 ml/hr.* How many micrograms per minute should the nurse administer?

12. For a postoperative patient who develops supraventricular tachycardia, the doctor prescribes a loading dose of esmolol hydrochloride (Brevibloc), followed by a maintenance dose of 5 g in 500 ml of D$_5$W, infused at 200 mcg/kg/min. The patient weighs 75 kg. What hourly flow rate should the nurse use to deliver the maintenance dose?

13. A patient with symptomatic bradycardia needs to receive 1 mg of isoproterenol hydrochloride (Isuprel) in 500 ml of D$_5$W, infused at 3 mcg/min. What hourly flow rate should the nurse use to administer this dose?

14. A patient on mechanical ventilation requires vecuronium bromide (Norcuron) to control respirations. So the doctor orders 20 mg of the drug in 100 ml of NS solution to infuse at 1 mcg/kg/min. The patient weighs 98 kg. At what hourly rate should the nurse set the infusion pump?

Answers to practice problems

◆ Calculating dosages for I.V. push drugs
1. 0.4 ml
2. 0.5 ml
3. 5 ml (1 ampule)
4. 0.75 ml
5. 2 ml

◆ Calculating I.V. flow rates
1. 8 ml/hr
2. 200 mcg/min
3. 75 ml/hr
4. 1 mg/min
5. 14 ml/hr; 71 ml/hr

Answers to review problems

1. 2 ml
2. 2.5 ml
3. 20 ml
4. 8 ml
5. 45 ml/hr
6. 5 mcg/kg/min
7. 1 mg
8. 10 ml/hr; 38 ml/hr
9. 2 mg/min
10. 2 mg/min
11. 50 mcg/min
12. 90 ml/hr
13. 90 ml/hr
14. 30 ml/hr

Comprehensive test

Answer the following questions about dosage calculations. To check your answers, see pages 269 through 274.

1. In the fraction $\frac{5}{7}$, which number is the numerator and which is the denominator?

2. Of the fractions $\frac{1}{4}$, $\frac{2}{3}$, and $\frac{10}{3}$, which is the improper fraction?

3. Reduce the following fractions to their lowest terms.

   a) $\frac{25}{50}$

   b) $\frac{3}{12}$

4. Of the numbers 5, 8, and 9, which one is a prime number?

5. For the fractions $\frac{1}{3}$, $\frac{1}{6}$, and $\frac{5}{8}$, what is the lowest common denominator?

6. Add the following sets of fractions.

   a) $\frac{1}{2} + \frac{2}{3} + \frac{1}{4}$

   b) $\frac{3}{4} + \frac{2}{7} + \frac{1}{8}$

   c) $\frac{1}{9} + \frac{2}{27} + \frac{1}{3}$

7. Subtract the following fractions.

   a) $\frac{7}{8} - \frac{3}{4}$

   b) $\frac{1}{2} - \frac{1}{3}$

8. Multiply the following fractions.

   a) $5\frac{2}{3} \times \frac{1}{4}$

   b) $\frac{2}{15} \times \frac{1}{2}$

9. Simplify the following complex fractions.

   a) $\dfrac{\frac{2}{3}}{\frac{3}{4}}$

   b) $\dfrac{\frac{1}{9}}{\frac{2}{12}}$

10. Divide the following fractions.

   a) $\dfrac{\frac{2}{3}}{1\frac{1}{3}}$

   b) $\dfrac{3\frac{1}{4}}{2\frac{2}{3}}$

11. In the following decimal fractions, what number is in the tenths place?

   a) 2.632

   b) 13.24

12. Round off the following decimal fractions to the nearest hundredth.

   a) 16.347

   b) 4.2689

13. Add the following decimal fractions.

   a) 2.389 + 0.6391

   b) 0.369 + 0.97 + 0.2

14. Subtract the following decimal fractions.

   a) 7.065 − 4.3

   b) 3.5 − 0.065

15. Multiply the following decimal fractions.

   a) 6.5 × 0.06

   b) 0.725 × 11.276

16. Convert the following decimal fractions to common fractions.

   a) 0.525

   b) 2.26

17. Convert the following percentages to decimal fractions.

   a) 75%

   b) 2.75%

18. Convert the following percentages to common fractions.

   a) 55%

   b) 23.5%

19. Convert the following common fractions to percentages.

   a) ⅖

   b) 5/12

20. What is 30% of 100?

21. What is 45% of 250?

22. 32 is what percent of 50?

23. What is 75% of 100?

24. Express the following ratios as fractions.

   a) 5 : 30

   b) The critical care unit has 5 registered nurses for every 10 patients.

25. Express the following numerical relationships in proportions with fractions.

   a) One tablet contains 325 mg of a drug; therefore, two tablets contain 650 mg.

   b) One ml of a solution contains 50 mg of a drug; therefore, 3 ml of the solution contains 150 mg.

26. Express the following numerical relationships in proportions with ratios.

   a) One ml of a solution contains 5 mg of a drug; therefore, 0.5 ml of the solution contains 2.5 mg.

   b) One case holds 12 bags of I.V. fluid; therefore, two cases hold 24 bags.

27. Solve for X in the following decimal fraction problems.

a) $X = \dfrac{0.3 \times 5}{0.05}$

b) $X = \dfrac{0.75 \times 2}{0.25}$

28. Solve for X in the following common fraction problems.

a) $X = \dfrac{\frac{1}{5} \times 3}{\frac{2}{5}}$

b) $X = \dfrac{\frac{3}{4} \times 4}{\frac{5}{8}}$

29. Solve for X in the following proportions, using ratios and fractions.

a) 3 : 15 :: X : 30

b) 1,000 : 10 :: 10,000 : X

c) $\dfrac{X}{50} = \dfrac{5}{25}$

d) $\dfrac{2}{5} = \dfrac{6}{X}$

30. The measurement system that includes grams, meters, and liters is the _____ system.

31. To convert milligrams to grams, move the decimal point _____ places to the _____ .

32. The abbreviation for microgram is _____ .

33. In the metric system, the basic unit used for measuring volume is the _____ .

34. In the metric system, the gram is the basic unit used to measure _____ .

35. Identify the proper abbreviations for the following metric measurements.

a) 37 micrograms

b) five-tenths of a milligram

c) 1,000 milliliters

36. The nurse can use a _____ _____ to measure volume in liters.

37. Perform the following metric conversions.

a) 1,500 ml = _____ L

b) 2,700 mcg = _____ mg

c) 5.4 g = _____ kg

d) 1,678 mcg = _____ mg

38. Add or subtract the following numbers and express the answer in grams.

a) 2 kg + 550 mg + 5 g

b) 4 g − 600 mg

39. Add or subtract the following numbers and express the answer in milliliters.

a) 200 ml + 0.25 L + 35 ml

b) 2 L − 750 ml − 25 ml

40. If the nurse removes 225 ml of a drug from a 2-liter bottle, how many milliliters should be left in the bottle?

41. If the nurse administers 250 mg of cefazolin sodium (Ancef) from a 1-g vial, how many milligrams should remain in the vial?

42. During an 8-hour shift, a patient received three I.V. drugs, each of which was mixed in 50 ml of fluid. The patient also received 700 ml of I.V. fluid. What is the patient's total I.V. intake in milliliters?

43. One phenobarbital (Luminal) tablet weighs 65 mg. How many milligrams do 12 tablets weigh?

44. In the apothecaries' system, the basic unit for measuring liquid volume is the

_____ .

45. Convert the following Arabic numbers to Roman numerals.

a) 7.5

b) 109

46. Convert the following Roman numerals to Arabic numbers.

a) vss

b) LXXXII

47. The doctor prescribes 1 fluidounce of acetaminophen (Tylenol) elixir P.O. for a patient. How many milliliters is this?

48. A patient must take 3 Tbs of a drug. How many teaspoons does this equal?

49. Perform the following conversions in the household measurement system.

a) 1 Tbs _____ gtt

b) ½ cup _____ Tbs

c) ½ tsp _____ gtt

d) 4 Tbs _____ tsp

50. A patient requires 18 units of insulin S.C. daily. How many milliliters of U-100 insulin should the patient receive?

51. The doctor orders 500,000 units of penicillin G for a patient. The pharmacy sends a vial labeled *penicillin G 200,000 U/ml.* How many milliliters should the nurse administer?

52. A patient who is receiving medications and feedings via a nasogastric tube needs to receive 10 mEq of potassium chloride (K-Dur). The label on the potassium container states *K-Dur potassium chloride, 30 mEq = 30 ml.* How many milliliters should the nurse give to the patient?

53. A patient who must restrict his fluid intake has been receiving 360 ml of fluid in each of the three food trays, daily. He must continue the same fluid restriction at home, where available containers are marked in ounces, pints, and quarts. How much fluid should the patient have at each meal?

54. While in the hospital, a child received 4 ml of a medication P.O. daily. At home, the child's parents will administer this medication, using a measuring device labeled in teaspoons. How many teaspoons of medication should the child receive?

55. Interpret the following drug orders.

a) nimodipine 60 mg P.O. q6h

b) Vasotec 1.25 mg I.V. q6h

c) 1,000 ml of D_5 ½NS I.V. with 20 mEq KCl at 125 ml/hr

d) phenytoin 1 g I.V. STAT

56. Write the following prescriptions as they would appear in a drug order.

a) Administer 5 mg of Compazine by intramuscular injection every 6 hours, as needed, for nausea and vomiting.

b) Administer a 650-mg acetaminophen suppository rectally every 4 hours, as needed for temperature greater than 101.5° F (measured rectally).

c) Immediately administer 10 units of regular insulin intravenously.

d) Discontinue the intravenous infusion of Isuprel.

57. Each drug order must contain the following information: date and time of the order, drug name, dosage form, _____ _____ , any restrictions or specifications related to the order, the doctor's signature, and the doctor's registration number for controlled drugs if applicable.

58. A medication administration record (MAR) reads *famotidine 20 mg I.V. q12h.* The last dose was given on Mar. 5 at 9 P.M. When should the nurse administer the next dose?

59. The nurse reviews an MAR, which states *gentamycin 80 mg I.V. q8h.* The patient received the last dose on Sept. 15 at 9 P.M. When should the nurse give the next dose?

60. A _____ -_____ pharmacy system immediately notifies the pharmacy of any changes in drug orders and decreases errors due to interpretation of handwriting.

61. Determine the division factor for I.V. administration sets with the following drip factors.

a) 10 gtt/ml

b) 60 gtt/ml

c) 15 gtt/ml

d) 20 gtt/ml

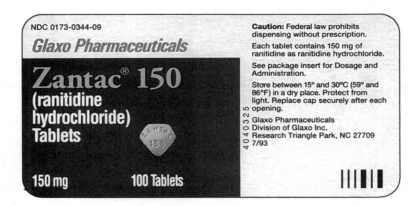

62. Based on the drug label above, answer the following questions.

   a) What is the trade name?

   b) What is the generic name?

   c) What is the dosage strength?

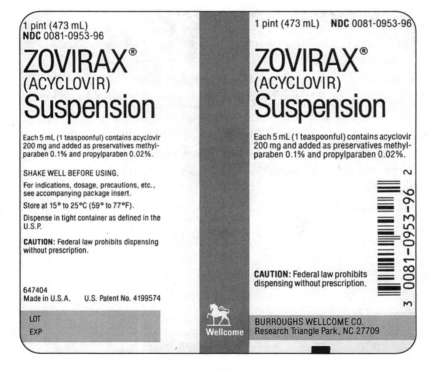

63. Based on the drug label above, answer the following questions.

   a) What is the trade name?

   b) What is the generic name?

   c) What is the dosage strength?

64. When pouring an oral solution into a medication cup, the nurse should hold the cup at

   _____ _____ .

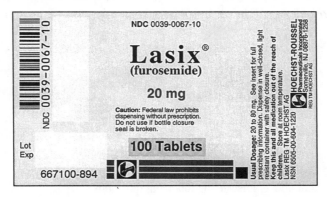

65 Based on the drug label above, perform the following dosage calculation.
The doctor prescribes glyburide (DiaBeta) 1.25 mg P.O. daily. How many tablets should the nurse administer to the patient?

66. Based on the drug label above, perform the following dosage calculation.
A patient needs to receive furosemide (Lasix) 80 mg P.O. daily. The pharmacy stocks Lasix in the dosage strength shown on the label above. How many tablets should the patient receive?

67. If propranolol hydrochloride (Inderal) is available in 60-mg tablets, but the drug order calls for a 90-mg dose, how many tablets should the nurse administer?

68. If digoxin (Lanoxin) is available in 0.25-mg tablets, but the drug order calls for an initial dose of 0.375 mg, how many tablets should the nurse administer?

69. The doctor prescribes levothyroxine sodium (Synthroid) 150 mcg P.O. daily. The pharmacy supplies 0.3-mg tablets of the drug. How many tablets should the nurse administer?

70. A geriatric patient cannot swallow a 160-mg tablet of furosemide (Lasix). To provide an equivalent dose, how many milliliters of 10 mg/ml-solution should the nurse administer?

71. A patient must receive theophylline (Elixophyllin) 200 mg P.O. b.i.d. The label on the Elixophyllin bottle indicates a concentration of 100 mg/5 ml. How many milliliters should the nurse administer with each dose?

72. The doctor prescribes amoxicillin trihydrate (Amoxil) 250 mg P.O. q8h. Amoxil is available in a 150-ml bottle that contains 250 mg/5 ml. How many doses does the bottle contain? How many days will it last?

73. A solution is a liquid preparation that contains a solute dissolved in a _____ .

74. _____ syringes have no dead space.

75. A _____ syringe holds up to 1 ml of medication and is used most frequently for intradermal injections.

76. A _____ syringe reduces medication errors and preparation time.

77. The doctor orders lorazepam (Ativan) 2 mg I.V. STAT. The drug is available in a prefilled syringe that contains a dosage strength of 1 mg/ml. How many milliliters of the drug should the nurse administer?

78. A patient needs to receive 100 mg of gentamicin sulfate (Garamycin) I.M. now, and a maintenance dose of 80 mg I.M. b.i.d. The drug comes in vials that contain 40 mg/ml. To the nearest tenth of a milliliter, how much should the nurse draw up for the initial dose? For the maintenance dose? What type of syringe should the nurse use to administer the drug?

79. What type of needle should *not* be used for injection?

80. A patient is to receive haloperidol (Haldol) 5 mg I.M. STAT for agitation. The label reads *Haldol haloperidol 5 mg/ml.* To what mark should the nurse fill a 3-ml syringe to administer this dose?

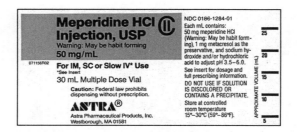

81. Based on the label above, answer the following questions.

    a) What is the generic name?

    b) What is the dosage strength?

    c) What is the total volume of this vial?

82. How many grams of dextrose are in 100 ml of a 50% dextrose solution?

83. The doctor prescribes 12.5 g of mannitol (Osmitrol) in a 25% solution I.V. q6h. How many milliliters should the nurse administer with each dose?

84. A vial of heparin sodium injection has a dosage strength of 10,000 U/ml. The total volume of the vial is 4 ml. The doctor prescribes heparin 25,000 U, added to an I.V. solution. How many milliliters of heparin should the nurse draw up to administer this dose?

85. A patient needs to receive 30 mEq of potassium chloride with his I.V. fluid. The drug vial contains 2 mEq/ml. How many milliliters should the nurse add to the I.V. fluid?

86. A drug label reads *sodium bicarbonate 8.4%, 50 mEq/50 ml, for slow intravenous use.* Each milliliter contains 84 mg of sodium bicarbonate. What is the dosage strength in mEq/ml? in mg/ml?

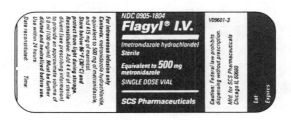

87. Based on the label above, answer the following questions.

a) What is the generic name?

b) How much diluent must be added to the vial for reconstitution?

c) What is the vial's total volume after drug reconstitution?

d) What is the drug's dosage strength?

e) If a patient needed to receive 250 mg of the drug, how many milliliters would the nurse withdraw from the vial?

f) The drug was reconstituted on Mar. 15 at 9 A.M. When will it expire?

88. After reconstituting a multiple-strength drug, the nurse must label the drug vial with what information?

89. If reconstitution information does not appear on the drug label, the nurse should check for it on the _____ _____ .

90. Regular insulin can be administered _____ to manage acute diabetic ketoacidosis.

91. The doctor orders 16 U of U-100 regular insulin S.C. STAT. The only syringe available is a 1-ml tuberculin syringe. How many milliliters should the nurse administer?

92. A patient needs to receive 45 U of U-100 NPH insulin S.C. daily. No insulin syringes are available. How many milliliters of insulin should the nurse administer via a 1-ml syringe?

93. A patient must receive 4 U of regular insulin S.C. STAT. What type of syringe should the nurse use to administer this dose?

94. A doctor's order states *15 U regular insulin, plus 40 U of NPH human insulin S.C. daily.* Based on this information, the nurse plans to use U-100 insulin. Which type of syringe should the nurse use? Which type of insulin should the nurse draw up first?

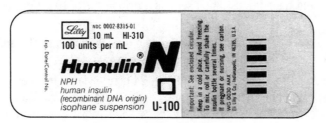

95. Based on the insulin label above, answer the following questions.

a) Before drawing up a dose of this insulin, the nurse should _____ the vial between the palms of the hands to mix it properly.

b) The doctor orders 35 U of NPH insulin S.C. q.a.m. How much insulin should the nurse draw up to administer this dose? What type of syringe should the nurse use?

c) The doctor orders 30 U of NPH insulin S.C. daily. No insulin syringes are available. How much insulin should the nurse draw up in a 1-ml syringe?

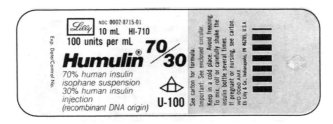

96. Based on the insulin label above, answer the following questions.

    a) The doctor orders 30 U of Humulin 70/30 insulin S.C. daily. To what mark on a U-100 syringe should the nurse draw up the insulin?

    b) If an insulin syringe were not available, to what mark on a tuberculin syringe would the nurse draw up the insulin?

97. A patient with acute diabetic ketoacidosis may require insulin via a continuous

_____ .

98. If a patient must receive 1,000 ml of D_5W over 24 hours through a microdrip set, what should the drip rate be?

99. A patient is to receive 500 ml of normal saline over 1 hour through an administration set with a drip factor of 15 gtt/ml. What should the drip rate be?

100. The doctor orders 50 ml of an I.V. drug to be given over 30 minutes. The nurse uses an administration set with a drip factor of 20 gtt/ml. What should the drip rate be?

101. A postoperative patient is to receive 3 L of dextrose 5% in normal saline over 24 hours. The administration set's drip factor is 15 gtt/ml. What should the drip rate be?

102. A patient must receive 1,000 ml of dextrose 5% in half normal saline over 10 hours. The administration set's drip factor is 10 gtt/ml. What is the drip rate? What is the 15-second count?

103. An I.V of 1,000 ml is infusing over 8 hours at 31 gtt/min, through an administration set with a drip factor of 15 gtt/ml. After 4 hours, the nurse notices 700 ml have been infused instead of 500 ml. How should the nurse adjust the drip rate for the remaining fluid?

104. A patient needs to receive 500 ml of 20% Liposyn I.V. over 12 hours via infusion pump. What hourly flow rate should the nurse set?

105. A patient needs to receive 1 unit of packed red blood cells over 3 hours. Each unit contains 250 ml, and the administration set has a drip factor of 10 gtt/ml. What should the drip rate be?

106. A patient must receive 100 ml of cryoprecipitate over 30 minutes. The administration set has a drip factor of 10 gtt/ml. What should the drip rate be?

107. A patient has been receiving 3 L of fluid over 24 hours, via an infusion pump that requires the nurse to set the hourly rate and volume. Now, the doctor writes a new order: *Decrease I.V. fluids to dextrose 5% in ¼NS, 2 L I.V. in 24 hours.* What were the pump settings for the original fluid order? How should the nurse set the pump for the new fluid order?

108. How long should it take to infuse 1 L of I.V. fluid at 100 ml/hr?

109. A patient is receiving an I.V. infusion of 1,000 ml of D_5W at 60 ml/hr. How long should it take to complete the infusion?

110. An I.V. of 500 ml of normal saline is infusing at 80 ml/hr. What is the total infusion time?

111. What is the total infusion time for 100 ml of D_5W infused at 6 gtt/min through an administration set with a drip factor of 15 gtt/ml?

112. A patient is receiving 1,000 ml of dextrose 5% in half normal saline at 31 gtt/min. The administration set's drip factor is 15 gtt/ml. If the infusion was started at 9 A.M., when will it be complete?

113. The doctor prescribes heparin sodium (Liquaemin Sodium) 25,000 U in 250 ml of D₅W to infuse at 1,600 U/hr. What flow rate should the nurse use to administer this dose?

114. A patient needs to receive 1,200 U/hr of heparin sodium (Liquaemin Sodium). Using a solution of 50,000 U in 500 ml of D₅W, the nurse should set the infusion pump at what flow rate?

115. A patient with acute diabetic ketoacidosis is to receive a continuous infusion of regular insulin 150 U in 150 ml of normal saline at 6 U/hr. What flow rate should the nurse set on the infusion pump?

116. A patient is receiving 150 U of insulin in 150 ml of normal saline I.V. at 10 ml/hr. How many units per hour is the patient receiving?

117. A patient must receive 1 L of total parenteral nutrition (TPN) solution over 24 hours. The administration set's drip factor is 15 gtt/ml. What should the flow rate be? What should the drip rate be?

118. An I.V. order states *2 L dextrose 5% in ½ NS I.V. over 24 hours. Add 1 vial of M.V.I.-12 to the first liter.* Each vial of M.V.I.-12 contains 5 ml of the drug. How many milliliters should the nurse add to the first liter of I.V. fluid?

119. A patient needs to receive 40 mEq of potassium chloride (K-Dur) in 1 L of D₅W. The electrolyte vial contains 2 mEq/ml. How many milliliters of potassium chloride should the nurse add?

120. A patient must receive 2.325 mEq of calcium gluconate (Kalcinate) I.V. in 1 L normal saline. The electrolyte dosage strength is 0.465 mEq/ml. How many milliliters should the nurse add to the I.V. fluid?

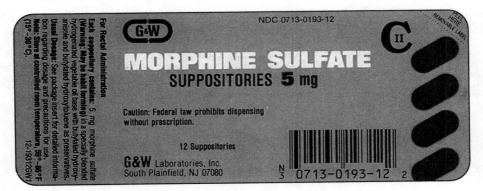

121. Based on the drug label above, answer the following questions.

    a) What is the drug's dosage strength?

    b) If the doctor prescribes morphine sulfate (Duramorph) 15 mg P.R. STAT, how many suppositories should the nurse administer?

    c) If the doctor prescribes morphine sulfate (Duramorph) 10 mg P.R. q4h p.r.n. pain, how many suppositories should the nurse administer with each dose?

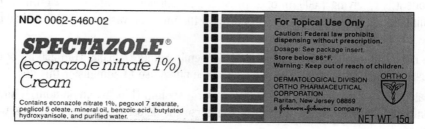

122. Based on the drug label above, answer the following questions.

a) What is the drug's trade name?

b) What is the drug's generic name?

123. Convert the following body weights to kilograms.

a) 65 lb

b) 35 lb

c) 8 lb

d) 27 lb

124. Using the body surface area (BSA) nomogram on page 223, determine the BSA for pediatric patients with the following characteristics.

a) 12 lb, 24″

b) 35 lb, 40 cm

c) 100 lb, 60″

d) 30 kg, 140 cm

125. If the pediatric dosage of amikacin sodium (Amikin) is 15 mg/kg/day P.O. divided b.i.d., how many milligrams should the nurse administer to a 6.5-kg infant every 12 hours?

126. If the pediatric dosage of phenytoin (Dilantin) suspension is 6 mg/kg/day P.O., how many milligrams should the nurse administer to a 21-kg child?

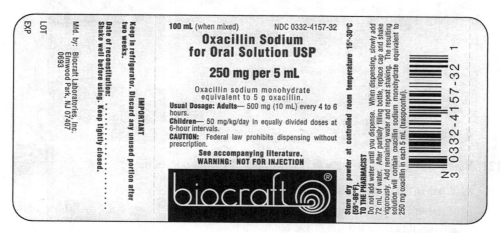

127. Based on the drug label above, perform the following dosage calculation. The doctor prescribes oxacillin sodium 80 mg P.O. q6h for a pediatric patient who weighs 12 kg. Is this dose within the usual dosage range?

128. The recommended pediatric dosage for ephedrine sulfate (Ephed II) is 100 mg/m²/day. For a child who weighs 12 lb and is 24″ tall, how much ephedrine should the nurse administer daily?

129. A 40-kg patient is to receive 8,000 mg of methicillin sodium (Staphcillin) I.V. daily in divided doses q6h. When diluted as directed on the drug label, the solution provides 1 g Staphcillin per 2 milliliters. How many milligrams should the patient receive with each dose? The recommended dosage range is 100 to 300 mg/kg I.V. daily. Does the prescribed dosage fall within the recommended range?

130. For a pediatric patient with a central line, the nurse should deliver a _____ -ml flush after administering medication through the line.

131. For a pediatric patient with a peripheral line, the nurse should deliver a _____ -ml flush after administering medication through the line.

132. A pediatric patient weighs 18 kg. How much fluid should the nurse administer over 24 hours to meet this child's basic fluid needs?

133. A pediatric patient requires 1,100 calories per day. What is this child's daily fluid requirement?

134. A pediatric patient has a BSA of 0.68 m². How much fluid does this child need every day?

135. What is the daily fluid requirement for a 5-year-old pediatric patient?

136. A solution contains 20 U of oxytocin in 1,000 ml normal saline. What is the solution's concentration in units per milliliter? What is its concentration in milliunits per milliliter?

137. The doctor prescribes magnesium sulfate 500 mg/hr I.V. A 1,000-ml bag contains 8 g of the drug. What is the solution's concentration in milligrams per milliliter? What should the flow rate be?

138. A major concern related to drug administration to a patient in labor is the drug's effects on the _____ .

139. The nurse should keep calcium gluconate (Kalcinate) on hand when administering _____ to a patient in labor.

140. A patient in preterm labor must receive ritodrine hydrochloride (Yutopar) 150 mg in 500 ml of D₅W I.V., starting at 100 mcg/min. What should the flow rate be?

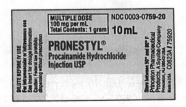

141. Based on the drug label above, perform the following dosage calculation.
For a patient with cardiac arrhythmias, the doctor prescribes procainamide hydrochloride (Pronestyl) 1 g in 250 ml of D₅W I.V., infused at 2 mg/min. What should the flow rate be?

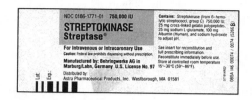

142. Based on the drug label above, perform the following dosage calculation.
A patient is to receive a loading dose of streptokinase (Streptase) 250,000 IU in 50 ml of normal saline I.V. to infuse over 30 minutes. To deliver this dose, what flow rate should the nurse set on the infusion pump?

143. If a solution contains 400 mg dopamine hydrochloride (Dopastat) in 250 ml D_5W, how many milligrams of dopamine should each milliliter of solution contain? How many micrograms is that?

144. A patient who weighs 65 kg must receive 5 mcg/kg/min of the above dopamine infusion. How many micrograms of dopamine should the patient receive each minute? What should the flow rate for 1 minute be? What hourly flow rate should the nurse set the infusion pump to deliver?

145. The doctor prescribes 50 mg of nitroprusside sodium (Nipride) mixed in 250 ml of D_5W. The patient weighs 70 kg and is to receive an infusion of 3 mcg/kg/min. What is the solution concentration? How many micrograms of nitroprusside should the patient receive each minute? What should the hourly flow rate be?

146. A patient is to receive 2 mg/min of bretylium tosylate (Bretylol) I.V. The solution contains 500 mg of bretylium in 50 ml of D_5W. What is the solution's concentration? How many milligrams should the patient receive each hour? What should the flow rate be?

147. The doctor prescribes lidocaine hydrochloride (Xylocaine) I.V. at 4 mg/min. The I.V. solution provides 2 g of lidocaine in 500 ml of D_5W. To infuse the drug at 4 mg/min, what should the flow rate per minute be? What should the hourly flow rate be?

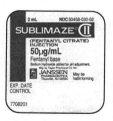

148. Based on the drug label above, perform the following dosage calculation.
Before inserting a central venous catheter, the doctor prescribes fentanyl citrate (Sublimaze) 100 mcg I.V. STAT. How many milliliters should the nurse administer?

Answers to comprehensive test

1. 5 is the numerator; 7 is the denominator.

2. $^{10}/_3$ is an improper fraction.

3. a) $\frac{1}{2}$

   b) $\frac{1}{4}$

4. 5 is a prime number.

5. 24 is the lowest common denominator.

6. a) $^{17}/_{12}$ or $1^5/_{12}$

   b) $1^9/_{56}$

   c) $^{14}/_{27}$

7. a) $\frac{1}{8}$

   b) $^1/_6$

8. a) $1^5/_{12}$

   b) $^1/_{15}$

9. a) $^8/_9$

   b) $^2/_3$

10. a) $\frac{1}{2}$

   b) $1^7/_{32}$

11. a) 6

   b) 2

12. a) 16.35

   b) 4.27

13. a) 3.0281

   b) 1.539

14. a) 2.765

   b) 3.435

15. a) 0.39

   b) 8.1751

16. a) $^{21}/_{40}$

   b) $2^{13}/_{50}$

17. a) 0.75

   b) 0.0275

18. a) $^{11}/_{20}$

   b) $^{47}/_{200}$

19. a) 40%

   b) 41.7%

20. 30

21. 112.5

22. 64%

23. 75

24. a) ⁵⁄₃₀ or ⅙

b) ⁵⁄₁₀ or ½

25. a) 1 tablet/325 mg = 2 tablets/650 mg

b) 1 ml/50 mg = 3 ml/150 mg

26. a) 1 : 5 :: 0.5 : 2.5

b) 1 : 12 :: 2 : 24

27. a) X = 30

b) X = 6

28. a) 1½

b) 4⅘

29. a) X = 6

b) X = 100

c) X = 10

d) X = 15

30. metric

31. three; left

32. mcg

33. liter

34. weight

35. a) 37 mcg

b) 0.5 mg

c) 1,000 ml

36. metric graduate

37. a) 1.5 L

b) 2.7 mg

c) 0.0054 kg

d) 1.678 mg

38. a) 2,005.55 g

b) 3.4 g

39. a) 485 ml

b) 1,225 ml

40. 1,775 ml

41. 750 mg

42. 850 ml

43. 780 mg

44. minim

45. a) viiss

b) CIX

46. a) 5.5

b) 82

47. 30 ml

48. 9 tsp

49. a) 180 gtt

b) 8 Tbs

c) 30 gtt

d) 12 tsp

50. 0.18 ml

51. 2.5 ml

52. 10 ml

53. 1½ cups or 12 oz

54. 1 tsp

55. a) Give 60 mg of nimodipine by mouth every 6 hours.

b) Give 1.25 mg of Vasotec I.V. every 6 hours.

c) Give 1,000 ml of dextrose 5% in half normal saline solution with 20 mEq of potassium chloride I.V. at 125 ml/hr.

d) Give 1 gram of phenytoin I.V. immediately.

56. a) Compazine 5 mg I.M. q6h p.r.n. N/V

b) acetaminophen supp. 650 mg P.R. q4h p.r.n. T > 101.5° F R

c) regular insulin 10 U I.V. STAT

d) D/C Isuprel I.V.

57. administration route

58. Mar. 6, 9 A.M.

59. Sept. 16, 5 A.M.

60. computer-based

61. a) 6

b) 1

c) 4

d) 3

62. a) Zantac

b) ranitidine hydrochloride

c) 150 mg

63. a) Zovirax Suspension

b) acyclovir

c) 200 mg/5 ml

64. eye level

65. ½ tablet

66. 4 tablets

67. 1½ tablets

68. 1½ tablets

69. ½ tablet

70. 16 ml

71. 10 ml

72. 30 doses; 10 days

73. solvent

74. Insulin

75. tuberculin

76. prefilled

77. 2 ml

78. 2.5 ml (initial dose); 2 ml (maintenance dose); a 3-ml standard syringe

79. filter needle

80. 1-ml mark

81. a) meperidine hydrochloride

   b) 50 mg/ml

   c) 30 ml

82. 50 grams

83. 50 ml

84. 2.5 ml

85. 15 ml

86. 1 mEq/ml; 84 mg/ml

87. a) metronidazole hydrochloride

   b) 4.4 ml

   c) 5 ml

   d) 100 mg/ml

   e) 2.5 ml

   f) Mar. 16 at 9 A.M.

88. The date and time of reconstitution and expiration, the nurse's initials (as the one who prepared the solution), and the dosage strength.

89. package insert

90. I.V.

91. 0.16 ml

92. 0.45 ml

93. low-dose insulin syringe

94. U-100 insulin syringe; regular insulin

95. a) roll

b) 35 units; U-100 insulin syringe

c) 0.3 ml

96. a) 30-U mark

b) 0.3-ml mark

97. I.V. infusion

98. 41.7 or 42 gtt/min

99. 125 gtt/min

100. 33.3 or 33 gtt/min

101. 31.3 or 31 gtt/min

102. 16.6 or 17 gtt/min; 4 gtt/15 sec

103. 18.75 or 19 gtt/min

104. 41.7 or 42 ml/hr

105. 13.9 or 14 gtt/min

106. 33.3 or 33 gtt/min

107. The original settings were 125 ml/hr (flow rate) and 1,000 ml (volume). The new settings should be 83 ml/hr (flow rate) and 1,000 ml (volume).

108. 10 hours

109. 16 hours, 40 minutes

110. 6 hours, 15 minutes

111. 4 hours, 10 minutes

112. 5:05 P.M.

113. 16 ml/hr

114. 12 ml/hr

115. 6 ml/hr

116. 10 U/hr

117. 41.7 or 42 ml/hr; 10.4 or 10 gtt/min

118. 5 ml

119. 20 ml

120. 5 ml

121. a) 5 mg/suppository

b) 3 suppositories

c) 2 suppositories

122. a) Spectazole

b) econazole nitrate

123. a) 29.5 or 30 kg

b) 15.9 or 16 kg

c) 3.6 kg or 4 kg

d) 12.3 or 12 kg

124. a) 0.32 m²

b) 0.68 m²

c) 1.42 m²

d) 1.08 m²

125. 48.75 or 49 mg

126. 126 mg

127. No, the recommended dosage is 50 mg/kg/day in divided doses q6h or 150 mg q6h.

128. 32 mg

129. 2,000 mg or 2 g; yes, because the range for a 40-kg patient is 4,000 to 12,000 mg daily.

130. 20 ml

131. 15 ml

132. 1,400 ml

133. 1,320 ml

134. 1,020 ml

135. 1,400 ml

136. 0.02 U/ml; 20 mU/ml

137. 8 mg/ml; 62.5 or 63 ml/hr

138. fetus

139. magnesium sulfate

140. 20 ml/hr

141. 30 ml/hr

142. 100 ml/hr

143. 1.6 mg/ml; 1,600 mcg/ml

144. 325 mcg/min; 0.2 ml/min; 12 ml/hr

145. 200 mcg/ml; 210 mcg/min; 63 ml/hr

146. 10 mg/ml; 120 mg/hr; 12 ml/hr

147. 1 ml/min; 60 ml/hr

148. 2 ml

Temperature conversions

When converting a patient's body temperature from Fahrenheit (F) to Celsius (C) or vice versa, use the following conversion formulas.

To convert Fahrenheit to Celsius:

$$(°F - 32) \times \tfrac{5}{9} = °C$$

To convert Celsius to Fahrenheit:

$$(°C \times \tfrac{9}{5}) + 32 = °F$$

The following examples show how to perform these conversions.

Suppose a temperature of 102° F needs to be converted to Celsius. The formula would look like this:

$$(102° F - 32) \times \tfrac{5}{9} = °C$$
$$70 \times \tfrac{5}{9} = °C$$
$$\tfrac{350}{9} = °C$$
$$38.9 = °C$$

Suppose a temperature of 35° C needs to be converted to Fahrenheit. The formula would look like this:

$$(35° C \times \tfrac{9}{5}) + 32 = °F$$
$$\tfrac{315}{5} + 32 = °F$$
$$63 + 32 = °F$$
$$95 = °F$$

For an even faster temperature conversion (rounded to the nearest tenth of a degree), use this table.

FAHRENHEIT DEGREES	CELSIUS DEGREES	FAHRENHEIT DEGREES	CELSIUS DEGREES
106.0	41.1	103.8	39.9
105.8	41.0	103.6	39.8
105.6	40.9	103.5	39.7
105.4	40.8	103.3	39.6
105.2	40.7	102.9	39.4
105.1	40.6	102.7	39.3
104.7	40.4	102.6	39.2
104.5	40.3	102.4	39.1
104.4	40.2	102.2	39.0
104.2	40.1	102.0	38.9
104.0	40.0	101.8	38.8

(continued)

Temperature conversions *(continued)*

FAHRENHEIT DEGREES	CELSIUS DEGREES	FAHRENHEIT DEGREES	CELSIUS DEGREES
101.7	38.7	95.7	35.4
101.5	38.6	95.5	35.3
101.1	38.4	95.4	35.2
100.9	38.3	95.2	35.1
100.8	38.2	95.0	35.0
100.6	38.1	94.8	34.9
100.4	38.0	94.6	34.8
100.2	37.9	94.5	34.7
100.0	37.8	94.3	34.6
99.9	37.7	93.9	34.4
99.7	37.6	93.7	34.3
99.3	37.4	93.6	34.2
99.1	37.3	93.4	34.1
99.0	37.2	93.2	34.0
98.8	37.1	93.0	33.9
98.6	37.0	92.8	33.8
98.4	36.9	92.7	33.7
98.2	36.8	92.5	33.6
98.1	36.7	92.1	33.4
97.9	36.6	91.9	33.3
97.5	36.4	91.8	33.2
97.3	36.3	91.6	33.1
97.2	36.2	91.4	33.0
97.0	36.1	91.2	32.9
96.8	36.0	91.0	32.8
96.6	35.9	90.9	32.7
96.4	35.8	90.7	32.6
96.2	35.7	90.3	32.4
96.1	35.6	90.1	32.3

Dimensional analysis

A variation of the proportion method with ratios, dimensional analysis (also known as factor analysis or factor labeling) is an alternative method of solving mathematical problems. Many nurses use dimensional analysis to calculate drug dosages because it eliminates the need to memorize formulas and requires only one equation to determine the answer. To compare the two methods at a glance, read the following problem and solutions.

The doctor prescribes 0.25 g of streptomycin sulfate I.M. The vial reads 2 ml = 1 g. How many milliliters should you administer?
Dimensional analysis

$$\frac{0.25 \text{ g}}{1} \times \frac{2 \text{ ml}}{1 \text{ g}} = 0.5 \text{ ml}$$

Proportion with ratios

$$1 \text{ g} : 2 \text{ ml} :: 0.25 \text{ g} : X \text{ ml}$$
$$X = 2 \times 0.25$$
$$X = 0.5 \text{ ml}$$

When using dimensional analysis, the nurse arranges a series of ratios, called factors, in a single (although sometimes lengthy) fractional equation. Each factor, written as a fraction, consists of two quantities and their units of measurement that are related to each other in a given problem. For instance, if 1,000 ml of a drug should be administered over 8 hours, the relationship between 1,000 ml and 8 hours is expressed by the fraction

$$\frac{1,000 \text{ ml}}{8 \text{ hr}}$$

When a problem includes a quantity and its unit of measurement that are unrelated to any other factor in the problem, they serve as the numerator of the fraction, and 1 (implied) becomes the denominator.

Some mathematical problems contain all of the information needed to identify the factors, set up the equation, and find the solution. Other problems require the use of a conversion factor. Conversion factors are equivalents (for example, 1 g = 1,000 mg) that the nurse can memorize or obtain from a conversion chart. Because the two quantities and units of measurement are equivalent, they can serve as the numerator or the denominator; thus, the conversion factor 1 g = 1,000 mg can be written in fraction form as

$$\frac{1,000 \text{ mg}}{1 \text{ g}} \quad \text{or} \quad \frac{1 \text{ g}}{1,000 \text{ mg}}$$

(continued)

Dimensional analysis *(continued)*

The factors given in the problem plus any conversion factors necessary to solve the problem are called *knowns*. The quantity of the answer, of course, is *unknown*. When setting up an equation in dimensional analysis, work backward, beginning with the unit of measurement of the answer. After plotting all the knowns, find the solution by following this sequence:

• Cancel similar quantities and units of measurement.

• Multiply the numerators.

• Multiply the denominators.

• Divide the numerator by the denominator.

Mastering dimensional analysis can take practice, but you may find your efforts well rewarded. To understand more fully how dimensional analysis works, review the following problem and the steps taken to solve it.

The doctor prescribes X grains (gr) of a drug. The pharmacy supplies the drug in 300-mg tablets (tab). How many tablets should you administer?

Write down the unit of measurement of the answer, followed by an "equal to" symbol (=).

$$tab =$$

Search the problem for the quantity with the same unit of measurement (if one doesn't exist, use a conversion factor). Place this in the numerator and its related quantity and unit of measurement in the denominator.

$$tab = \frac{1 \; tab}{300 \; mg}$$

Separate the first factor from the next with a multiplication symbol (×).

$$tab = \frac{1 \; tab}{300 \; mg} \times$$

Place the unit of measurement of the denominator of the first factor in the numerator of the second factor; search the problem for the quantity with the same unit of measurement (if one doesn't exist, as in this example, use a conversion factor); place this in the numerator and its related quantity and unit of measurement in the denominator, and follow with a multiplication symbol. Repeat this step until all known factors are included in the equation.

$$tab = \frac{1 \; tab}{300 \; mg} \times \frac{60 \; mg}{1 \; gr} \times \frac{10 \; gr}{1}$$

Dimensional analysis (continued)

Treat the equation as a large fraction. First, cancel similar units of measurement in the numerator and the denominator. What remains should be what you began with—the unit of measurement of the answer. If not, recheck your equation to find and correct the error. Next, multiply the numerators and then the denominators. Finally, divide the numerator by the denominator.

$$\text{tab} = \frac{1 \text{ tab}}{300 \text{ mg}} \times \frac{60 \text{ mg}}{1 \text{ gr}} \times \frac{10 \text{ gr}}{1}$$

$$= \frac{60 \times 10 \text{ tab}}{300}$$

$$= \frac{600 \text{ tab}}{300}$$

$$= 2 \text{ tablets}$$

For additional practice, study the following examples, which use dimensional analysis to solve various mathematical problems common to dosage calculations and drug administration.

1. *A patient weighs 140 lb. What is his weight in kilograms (kg)?*

Unit of measurement of the answer: kg

$$\text{1st factor (conversion factor): } \frac{1 \text{ kg}}{2.2 \text{ lb}}$$

$$\text{2nd factor: } \frac{140 \text{ lb}}{1}$$

$$\text{kg} = \frac{1 \text{ kg}}{2.2 \text{ lb}} \times 140 \text{ lb}$$

$$= \frac{140 \text{ kg}}{2.2}$$

$$= 63.6 \text{ kg}$$

2. *The doctor prescribes 75 mg of a drug. The pharmacy stocks a multidose vial containing 100 mg/ml. How many milliliters should the nurse administer?*

Unit of measurement of the answer: ml

$$\text{1st factor: } \frac{1 \text{ ml}}{100 \text{ mg}}$$

$$\text{2nd factor: } \frac{75 \text{ mg}}{1}$$

$$\text{ml} = \frac{1 \text{ ml}}{100 \text{ mg}} \times \frac{75 \text{ mg}}{1}$$

$$= \frac{75 \text{ ml}}{100}$$

$$= 0.75 \text{ ml}$$

(continued)

Dimensional analysis *(continued)*

3. *The doctor prescribes 1 teaspoon (tsp) of a cough elixir. The pharmacist sends up a bottle whose label reads 1 ml = 50 mg. How many milligrams should the nurse administer?*

Unit of measurement of the answer: mg

$$\text{1st factor: } \frac{50 \text{ mg}}{1 \text{ ml}}$$

$$\text{2nd factor (conversion factor): } \frac{5 \text{ ml}}{1 \text{ tsp}}$$

$$\text{3rd factor: } \frac{1 \text{ tsp}}{1}$$

$$\text{mg} = \frac{50 \text{ mg}}{1 \text{ ml}} \times \frac{5 \text{ ml}}{1 \text{ tsp}} \times \frac{1 \text{ tsp}}{1}$$

$$= 50 \text{ mg} \times \frac{5}{1}$$

$$= 250 \text{ mg}$$

4. *The doctor prescribes 1,000 ml of an I.V. solution to be administered over 8 hours. The I.V. tubing delivers 15 gtt/ml/min. What is the infusion rate in gtt/min?*

Unit of measurement of the answer: gtt/min

$$\text{1st factor: } \frac{15 \text{ gtt}}{1 \text{ ml}}$$

$$\text{2nd factor: } \frac{1,000 \text{ ml}}{8 \text{ hr}}$$

$$\text{3rd factor (conversion factor): } \frac{1 \text{ hr}}{60 \text{ min}}$$

$$\text{gtt/min} = \frac{15 \text{ gtt}}{1 \text{ ml}} \times \frac{1,000 \text{ ml}}{8 \text{ hr}} \times \frac{1 \text{ hr}}{60 \text{ min}}$$

$$= \frac{15 \text{ gtt} \times 1,000 \times 1}{8 \times 60 \text{ min}}$$

$$= \frac{15,000 \text{ gtt}}{480 \text{ min}}$$

$$= 31.3 \text{ or } 31 \text{ gtt/min}$$

Dimensional analysis *(continued)*

5. The doctor prescribes 10,000 units (U) of heparin added to 500 ml of 5% dextrose in water at 1,200 U/hr. How many drops per minute should the nurse administer if the I.V. tubing delivers 10 gtt/ml?
Unit of measurement of the answer: gtt/min

$$\text{1st factor: } \frac{10 \text{ gtt}}{1 \text{ ml}}$$

$$\text{2nd factor: } \frac{500 \text{ ml}}{10,000 \text{ U}}$$

$$\text{3rd factor: } \frac{1,200 \text{ U}}{1 \text{ hr}}$$

$$\text{4th factor (conversion factor): } \frac{1 \text{ hr}}{60 \text{ min}}$$

$$\text{gtt/min} = \frac{10 \text{ gtt}}{1 \text{ ml}} \times \frac{500 \text{ ml}}{10,000 \text{ U}} \times \frac{1,200 \text{ U}}{1 \text{ hr}} \times \frac{1 \text{ hr}}{60 \text{ min}}$$

$$= \frac{10 \times 500 \times 1,200 \text{ gtt}}{10,000 \times 60 \text{ min}}$$

$$= \frac{6,000,000 \text{ gtt}}{600,000 \text{ min}}$$

$$= 10 \text{ gtt/min}$$

◆ Practice problems

1. A pediatric patient weighs 32 kg. What is the child's weight in pounds (lb)?

2. The doctor orders diphenhydramine hydrochloride 25 mg I.V. t.i.d. The pharmacy supplies the drug in a vial that contains 50 mg/ml. How many milliliters of the drug should the nurse administer?

3. The pediatrician prescribes acetaminophen elixir 2 tsp every 4 to 6 hours. The pharmacist provides a bottle containing 160 mg/5 ml. How many milligrams should the nurse administer?

4. The doctor prescribes D_5 ½ NSS 1,000 ml I.V. to be infused over 6 hours. The I.V. tubing delivers 10 gtt/ml/min. What is the drip rate in gtt/min?

5. The doctor prescribes heparin 25,000 U I.V., added to 250 ml of D_5W and infused at 1,600 U/hr. How many drops should the nurse administer if the I.V. tubing delivers 15 gtt/ml?

(continued)

Dimensional analysis *(continued)*

◆ Answers to practice problems

1.
$$1\text{st factor: } \frac{2.2 \text{ lb}}{1 \text{ kg}}$$

$$2\text{nd factor: } \frac{32 \text{ kg}}{1}$$

$$\text{lb} = \frac{2.2 \text{ lb}}{1 \text{ kg}} \times \frac{32 \text{ kg}}{1}$$

$$= 2.2 \text{ lb} \times 32$$

$$= 70.4 \text{ lb}$$

2.
$$1\text{st factor: } \frac{1 \text{ ml}}{50 \text{ mg}}$$

$$2\text{nd factor: } \frac{25 \text{ mg}}{1}$$

$$\text{ml} = \frac{1 \text{ ml}}{50 \text{ mg}} \times \frac{25 \text{ mg}}{1}$$

$$= \frac{25 \text{ ml}}{50}$$

$$= 0.5 \text{ ml}$$

3.
$$1\text{st factor: } \frac{160 \text{ mg}}{5 \text{ ml}}$$

$$2\text{nd factor: } \frac{5 \text{ ml}}{1 \text{ tsp}}$$

$$3\text{rd factor: } \frac{2 \text{ tsp}}{1}$$

$$\text{mg} = \frac{160 \text{ mg}}{5 \text{ ml}} \times \frac{5 \text{ ml}}{1 \text{ tsp}} \times \frac{2 \text{ tsp}}{1}$$

$$= \frac{1{,}600 \text{ mg}}{5}$$

$$= 320 \text{ mg}$$

Dimensional analysis *(continued)*

4.

1st factor: $\dfrac{10 \text{ gtt}}{1 \text{ ml}}$

2nd factor: $\dfrac{1,000 \text{ ml}}{6 \text{ hr}}$

3rd factor: $\dfrac{1 \text{ hr}}{60 \text{ min}}$

$$\text{gtt/min} = \frac{10 \text{ gtt}}{1 \text{ ml}} \times \frac{1,000 \text{ ml}}{6 \text{ hr}} \times \frac{1 \text{ hr}}{60 \text{ min}}$$

$$= \frac{10 \text{ gtt} \times 1,000 \times 1}{6 \times 60 \text{ min}}$$

$$= \frac{10,000 \text{ gtt}}{360 \text{ min}}$$

$$= 27.7 \text{ or } 28 \text{ gtt/min}$$

5.

1st factor: $\dfrac{15 \text{ gtt}}{1 \text{ ml}}$

2nd factor: $\dfrac{250 \text{ ml}}{25,000 \text{ U}}$

3rd factor: $\dfrac{1,600 \text{ U}}{1 \text{ hr}}$

4th factor: $\dfrac{1 \text{ hr}}{60 \text{ min}}$

$$\text{gtt/min} = \frac{15 \text{ gtt}}{1 \text{ ml}} \times \frac{250 \text{ ml}}{25,000 \text{ U}} \times \frac{1,600 \text{ U}}{1 \text{ hr}} \times \frac{1 \text{ hr}}{60 \text{ min}}$$

$$= \frac{15 \times 250 \times 1,600 \text{ gtt}}{25,000 \times 60 \text{ min}}$$

$$= \frac{6,000,000 \text{ gtt}}{1,500,000 \text{ min}}$$

$$= 4 \text{ gtt/min}$$

APPENDIX C

Equations for selected drug calculations

PEDIATRIC DOSAGES

Based on weight (in kilograms)

$$\text{Child's drug dosage} = \text{Child's weight (kg)} \times \frac{\text{Drug dosage (mg)}}{1 \text{ kg}}$$

Based on body surface area (BSA)

$$\text{Child's drug dosage} = \text{Child's BSA (m}^2) \times \frac{\text{Drug dose (mg)}}{1 \text{ m}^2}$$

Based on an adult dose

$$\text{Child's drug dosage} = \frac{\text{Child's BSA}}{\underset{(1.73 \text{ m}^2)}{\text{Average adult BSA}}} \times \text{Average adult dose (mg)}$$

PEDIATRIC FLUID NEEDS

Based on weight (in kilograms)

Up to 10 kg

$$\text{Fluid requirements (ml/24 hr)} = \text{Child's weight (kg)} \times 100 \text{ ml/kg}$$

Between 10 and 20 kg

$$\text{Fluid requirements (ml/24 hr)} = 1{,}000 \text{ ml} + (50 \text{ ml} \times \text{weight over 10 kg})$$

Over 20 kg

$$\text{Fluid requirements (ml/24 hr)} = 1{,}500 \text{ ml} + (20 \text{ ml} \times \text{weight over 20 kg})$$

Based on calories of metabolism

$$\text{Fluid requirements (ml/24 hr)} = \frac{\text{Calorie requirements}}{100} \times 120 \text{ ml/kcal}$$

Based on BSA

$$\text{Maintenance fluid requirements (ml/24 hr)} = \text{BSA (m}^2) \times 1{,}500 \text{ ml/day/m}^2$$

Based on age

Less than age 1 (requires 125 to 150 ml/kg)

$$\text{Lower boundary (ml/24 hr)} = \text{Child's weight (kg)} \times 125 \text{ ml/kg}$$

$$\text{Upper boundary (ml/24 hr)} = \text{Child's weight (kg)} \times 150 \text{ ml/kg}$$

Age 1 or older (requires 1,000 ml plus 100 ml for each year above age 1; not to exceed 2,500 ml/24 hr)

$$\text{Fluid requirements (ml/24 hr)} = 1{,}000 \text{ ml} + (50 \text{ ml} \times \text{age} > 1 \text{ year})$$

APPENDIX C

Equations for selected drug calculations (continued)

I.V. SOLUTIONS

Concentration

$$\frac{\text{mg of medication}}{\text{ml of I.V. fluid}} = \text{Concentration (mg/ml)}$$

Flow rate

Flow rate per minute

$$\frac{\text{Dose per minute}}{\text{X ml/minute}} = \frac{\text{Concentration of solution}}{1 \text{ ml of I.V. fluid}}$$

Hourly flow rate

Step 1:

Hourly dosage = Ordered dosage (mcg/min) × 60 min

Step 2:

$$\frac{\text{Hourly dosage}}{\text{X ml}} = \frac{\text{Concentration of solution}}{1 \text{ ml of I.V. fluid}}$$

Drip rates

For microdrip sets

Drip rate = Flow rate

For sets with a drip factor of 10

$$\text{Drip rate} = \frac{\text{Flow rate}}{6}$$

For sets with a drip factor of 15

$$\text{Drip rate} = \frac{\text{Flow rate}}{4}$$

For sets with a drip factor of 20

$$\text{Drip rate} = \frac{\text{Flow rate}}{3}$$

Ensuring safe I.V. dosages

Given the amount of medication to be placed in a particular type and volume of I.V. solution and the hourly flow rate for the solution, the nurse must determine whether the amount administered (in mg/kg/minute) is a safe and effective dosage.

♦ Determine the concentration of the solution.

♦ Determine the amount of medication being administered each hour and each minute.

Each hour

> Flow rate × Solution concentration = Medication received (mg/hour)

Each minute

$$\frac{\text{Medication received (mg/hour)}}{60 \text{ min/hour}} = \text{Medication received (mg/minute)}$$

♦ Determine the amount of medication received each minute per kilogram of patient body weight.

$$\frac{\text{Medication received (mg/minute)}}{\text{Patient's weight (kg)}} = \text{mg/kg/minute}$$

♦ Compare the amount of medication being received by the patient (mg/kg/minute) to the dosage recommended in a resource text.

Reporting medication errors

Medication errors can occur for various reasons, such as lack of knowledge about drug administration, incorrect dosage calculations, and transcription errors. To help identify causes of errors—and help prevent them in the future—the United States Pharmacopeia (USP) Medication Error Reporting Program tracks medication errors across the country.

If you make a medication error, simply report it to the program by calling the toll-free telephone number or by sending a completed copy of the form shown below. Then the USP will forward the information to the Food and Drug Administration, the product manufacturer or labeler, and the Institute for Safe Medication Practices. When this information is compiled, it is used to spot trends and possible causes of errors, such as product labeling, so that they can be corrected. (For blank copies of the form, call 1-800-23-ERROR.)

MEDICATION ERRORS REPORTING PROGRAM

USP MEDICATION ERRORS REPORTING PROGRAM
Presented in cooperation with the Institute for Safe Medication Practices
The USP Practitioners' Reporting Network℠ is an FDA MEDWATCH partner

❑ ACTUAL ERROR   ❑ POTENTIAL ERROR

Please describe the error. Include sequence of events, personnel involved, and work environment (e.g., code situation, change of shift, short staffing, no 24-hr. pharmacy, floor stock). If more space is needed, please attach separate page.

Was the medication administered to or used by the patient? ❑ No ❑ Yes   Date and time of event: _____

What type of staff or health care practitioner made the initial error? _____

Describe outcome (e.g., death, type of injury, adverse reaction). _____

If the medication did not reach the patient, describe the intervention. _____

Who discovered the error? _____

When and how was error discovered? _____

Where did the error occur (e.g., hospital, outpatient or retail pharmacy, nursing home, patient's home)? _____

Was another practitioner involved in the error? ❑ No ❑ Yes If yes, what type of practitioner? _____

Was patient counseling provided? ❑ No ❑ Yes If yes, before or after error was discovered? _____

If a product was involved, please complete the following:

	Product #1	Product #2
Brand name of product involved		
Generic name		
Manufacturer		
Labeler (if different from mfr.)		
Dosage form		
Strength/concentration		
Type and size of container		
NDC number		

If available, please provide relevant patient information (age, gender, diagnosis, etc.). Patient identification not required.

Reports are most useful when relevant materials such as product label, copy of prescription/order, etc. can be reviewed.
Can these materials be provided? ❑ No ❑ Yes If yes, please specify. _____

Suggest any recommendations you have to prevent recurrence of this error or describe policies or procedures you have instituted to prevent future similar errors.

A copy of this report is routinely sent to the Institute for Safe Medication Practices (ISMP), to the manufacturer/labeler, and to the Food and Drug Administration (FDA). **USP may release my identity to: (check boxes that apply)**
❑ ISMP ❑ The manufacturer and/or labeler as listed above ❑ FDA ❑ Other persons requesting a copy of this report ❑ Anonymous to all

Your name and title

Your facility name, address, and ZIP

Telephone number (include area code)

Signature

Date

Return to the attention of:
Diane D. Cousins, R.Ph.
USP PRN
12601 Twinbrook Parkway
Rockville, MD 20852-1790

Call Toll Free: **800-23-ERROR** (800-233-7767)
or FAX 301-816-8532

Electronic reporting forms are available. Please call for additional information and/or your free diskette.

Date Received by USP:

File Access Number:

C-194

Additional forms can be found in the *USP DI Vol. I* and *Vol. III* and in all monthly *Updates*.

APPENDIX F

Drugs that must not be crushed

When you are preparing solid drugs for administration, be careful not to crush or dissolve a drug if doing so can impair its effectiveness or absorption. Many drug forms (such as slow-release, enteric-coated, encapsulated-bead, wax-matrix, sublingual, or buccal preparations) are formulated to release their active ingredient for a specified duration or at a predetermined time after administration. Disrupting these formulations by crushing can dramatically affect the drug absorption rate and increase the risk of adverse effects.

Other reasons not to crush a specific drug form involve such considerations as taste, tissue irritation, and unusual formulation—for example, a capsule within a capsule, a liquid within a capsule, or a multiple, compressed tablet.

Avoid crushing these drugs, which are listed here by brand name, for the reasons noted beside them.

Accutane (mucous membrane irritant)
Actifed 12-Hour (slow release)
Acutrim (slow release)
Adipost capsules (slow release)
Aerolate SR, JR, III (slow release)
Afrinol Repetabs (slow release)
Aller-Chlor (slow release)
Allerest 12-Hour (slow release)
Ammonium Chloride Enseals (enteric coated)
APF Arthritis Pain Formula (enteric coated)
Artane Sequels (slow release)
ASA Enseals (enteric coated)
Atrohist LA, Sprinkle (slow release)
Azulfidine EN-Tabs (enteric coated)
Bayer Timed-Release Arthritic Pain Formula (slow release)
Belladenal S (slow release)
Bellergal S (slow release)
Betapen VK (taste)
Bisacodyl (enteric coated)
Bisco-Lax (enteric coated)
Bontril Slow-Release (slow release)
Breonesin (liquid filled)
Brexin LA (slow release)
Bromfed (slow release)
Bromfed PD (slow release)
Bromphen (slow release)
Bromphen TD (slow release)
Calan SR (slow release)
Carbiset TR (slow release)

Cardizem (slow release)
Cardizem CD, SR (slow release)
Carter's Little Pills (enteric coated)
Ceftin (taste)
Cerespan (slow release)
Charcoal Plus (enteric coated)
Chloral Hydrate (liquid within a capsule, taste)
Chlorpheniramine Maleate Time Release (slow release)
Chlor-Trimeton Decongestant Repetabs (slow release)
Chlor-Trimeton Repetabs (slow release)
Choledyl (enteric coated)
Choledyl SA (slow release)
Cipro (taste)
Codimal LA (slow release)
Colace (liquid within a capsule, taste)
Comhist LA (slow release)
Compazine Spansules (slow release)
Congess SR, JR (slow release)
Constant T (slow release)
Contac 12-Hour, Maximum Strength (slow release)
Control (slow release)
Cotazym S (enteric coated)
Creon (enteric coated)
Cystospaz M (slow release)
Dallergy (slow release)
Dallergy D, JR (slow release)
Deconamine SR (slow release)
Deconsal LA, Sprinkle, II (slow release)

Drugs that must not be crushed *(continued)*

Depakene (slow release, mucous
 membrane irritant)
Dehist (slow release)
Demazin Repetabs (slow release)
Depakote (enteric coated)
Desoxyn Gradumet (slow release)
Desyrel (taste)
Dexatrim (slow release)
Dexedrine Spansules (slow release)
Diamox Sequels (slow release)
Diethylstilbestrol Enseals (enteric coated)
Dilatrate SR (slow release)
Dimetane Extentabs (slow release)
Dimetapp Extentabs (slow release)
Disobrom (slow release)
Donnatal Extentabs (slow release)
Donnazyme (slow release)
Drisdol (liquid filled)
Drixoral (slow release)
Drixoral Sinus (slow release)
Drize (slow release)
Dulcolax (enteric coated)
Duotrate (slow release)
Duraquin (slow release)
Easprin (enteric coated)
Ecotrin (enteric coated)
Ecotrin Maximum Strength (enteric
 coated)
E.E.S. 400 Filmtab (enteric coated)
Elixophyllin SR (slow release)
E-Mycin (enteric coated)
Endafed (slow release)
Entex LA (slow release)
Entozyme (enteric coated)
Equanil (taste)
Ergostat (sublingual)
Eryc (enteric coated)
Ery-Tab (enteric coated)
Erythrocin Stearate (enteric coated)
Erythromycin Base (enteric coated)
Eskalith CR (slow release)
Extendryl SR, JR (slow release)
Fedahist Gyrocaps, Timecaps (slow
 release)
Feldene (mucous membrane irritant)
Feocyte (slow release)

Feosol (enteric coated)
Feosol Spansules (slow release)
Feratab (enteric coated)
Fergon (slow release)
Fero-Grad 500 mg (slow release)
Fero-Gradumet (slow release)
Ferralet SR (slow release)
Ferralyn Lanacap (slow release)
Ferro-Sequel (slow release)
Ferrous Sulfate Enseals (enteric coated)
Festal II (enteric coated)
Feverall Sprinkle Caps (taste)
Fumatinic (slow release)
Genabid (slow release)
Geocillin (taste)
Gris-PEG (crushing may cause
 precipitation as larger particles)
Guaifed (slow release)
Guaifed PD (slow release)
Hispril Spansules (slow release)
Histaspan D, Plus (slow release)
Humibid Sprinkle, DM, DM Sprinkle, LA
 (slow release)
Hydergine LC (liquid within a capsule)
Hydergine Sublingual (sublingual)
Hytakerol (liquid filled)
Iberet (slow release)
Iberet 500 (slow release)
Ilotycin (enteric coated)
Inderal LA (slow release)
Inderide LA (slow release)
Indocin SR (slow release)
Ionamin (slow release)
Iso-Bid (slow release)
Isoclor Timesules (slow release)
Isoptin SR (slow release)
Isordil Sublingual (sublingual)
Isordil Tembids (slow release)
Isosorbide Dinitrate SR (slow release)
Isosorbide Dinitrate Sublingual
 (sublingual)
Isuprel Glossets (sublingual)
Kaon Cl (slow release)
K-Dur (slow release)
Klor-Con (slow release)
Klotrix (slow release)

(continued)

Drugs that must not be crushed *(continued)*

K-Tab (slow release)
K + 10 (slow release)
Levsinex Timecaps (slow release)
Levsinex with Pb Timecaps (slow release)
Lithobid (slow release)
Mandameth (enteric coated)
Measurin (slow release)
Meprospan (slow release)
Mestinon Timespans (slow release)
Mi-Cebrin (enteric coated)
Mi-Cebrin T (enteric coated)
Micro-K (slow release)
Micro-K Extencaps (slow release)
Motrin (taste)
MS Contin (slow release)
Naldecon (slow release)
Niac (slow release)
Nico 400 (slow release)
Nicobid (slow release)
Nicobid Tempules (slow release)
Nitro-Bid (slow release)
Nitro-Bid Plateau Caps (slow release)
Nitrocine Timecaps (slow release)
Nitroglyn (slow release)
Nitrong (sublingual)
Nitrospan (slow release)
Nitrostat (sublingual)
Nitrostat SR (slow release)
Noctec (liquid within a capsule)
Nolamine (slow release)
Nolex LA (slow release)
Norflex (slow release)
Norpace CR (slow release)
Novafed (slow release)
Novafed A (slow release)
Optilets 500 Filmtab (enteric coated)
Optilets M 500 Filmtab (enteric coated)
Oramorph SR (slow release)
Orflagen (slow release)
Ornade Spansules (slow release)
Pabalate (enteric coated)
Pabalate SF (enteric coated)
Pancrease (enteric coated)
Pancrease MT (enteric coated)
Pancreatin Enseals Triple Strength (enteric coated)

Papaverine Sustained Action (slow release)
Pathilon Sequels (slow release)
Pavabid Plateau Caps (slow release)
PBZ SR (slow release)
PCE (slow release)
Pentol SA (slow release)
Perdiem (wax coated)
Peritrate SA (slow release)
Permitil Chronotab (slow release)
Phazyme (slow release)
Phazyme 95 (slow release)
Phenergan (taste)
Phenetron Compound (enteric coated)
Phyllocontin (slow release)
Plendil (slow release)
Polaramine Repetabs (slow release)
Poly-Histine D (slow release)
Potassium Chloride Enseals (enteric coated)
Potassium Iodide Enseals (enteric coated)
Prelu 2 (slow release)
Preludin Enduret (slow release)
Prilosec (slow release)
Pro-Banthine (taste)
Procainamide HCL SR (slow release)
Procan SR (slow release)
Procardia (delays absorption)
Procardia XL (slow release)
Promine SR (slow release)
Pronestyl SR (slow release)
Proventil Repetabs (slow release)
Prozac (slow release)
Quadra Hist (slow release)
Quibron Bidcaps (slow release)
Quibron-T/SR (slow release)
Quinaglute Dura-tabs (slow release)
Quinalan Lanatabs, SR (slow release)
Quinidex Extentabs (slow release)
Respaire SR (slow release)
Respbid (slow release)
Ritalin SR (slow release)
Robimycin Robitab (enteric coated)
Rondec TR (slow release)
Roxanol SR (slow release)
Ru-Tuss (slow release)

APPENDIX F

Drugs that must not be crushed *(continued)*

Ru-Tuss DE, II (slow release)
Sinemet CR (slow release)
Singlet (slow release)
Slo-bid Gyrocaps (slow release)
Slo-Niacin (slow release)
Slo-Phyllin GG, Gyrocaps (slow release)
Slow-Fe (slow release)
Slow-K (slow release)
Slow-Mag (slow release)
Sodium Chloride Enseals (enteric coated)
Sodium Salicylate Enseals (enteric coated)
Somophyllin CRT (slow release)
Sorbitrate SA (slow release)
Sorbitrate Sublingual (sublingual)
Span-FF (slow release)
Sparine (taste)
S-P-T (liquid gelatin suspension)
Sudafed 12-Hour (slow release)
Sustaire (slow release)
Tamine SR (slow release)
Tavist D (multiple compressed tablet)
Tedral SA (slow release)
Teldrin (slow release)
Teldrin Spansules (slow release)
Temaril Spansules (slow release)
Ten-K (slow release)
Tenuate Dospan (slow release)
Tepanil Ten-Tab (slow release)
Tessalon Perles (slow release)
Theobid (slow release)
Theobid Duracap, JR Duracap (slow release)
Theochron (slow release)
Theoclear LA (slow release)
Theo-Dur (slow release)

Theo-Dur Sprinkle (slow release)
Theolair SR (slow release)
Theo-Sav (slow release)
Theospan SR (slow release)
Theo-Time (slow release)
Theo-24 (slow release)
Theovent (slow release)
Theox (slow release)
Therapy Bayer (enteric coated)
Thorazine Spansules (slow release)
Thyroid Enseals (enteric coated)
Toprol XL (slow release)
T-Phyl (slow release)
Tranxene SD (slow release)
Trental (slow release)
Triaminic (slow release)
Triaminic TR (slow release)
Triaminic 12 (slow release)
Trilafon Repetabs (slow release)
Trinalin Repetabs (slow release)
Triptone Caplets (slow release)
Tuss LA (slow release)
Tuss-Ornade Spansules (slow release)
ULR LA (slow release)
Uniphyl (slow release)
Uracel 5 (enteric coated)
Valrelease (slow release)
Verelan (slow release)
Verin (slow release)
Voltaren (enteric coated)
Wellbutrin (mucous membrane anesthetic)
Wyamycin S (slow release)
Wygesic (taste)
ZORprin (slow release)
Zymase (enteric coated)

Selected references

Baer, C., and Williams, B. *Clinical Pharmacology and Nursing,* 3rd ed. Springhouse, Pa.: Springhouse Corp., 1996.

Bobak, I., et al. *Maternity Nursing,* 4th ed. St. Louis: Mosby-Year Book, 1995.

Hudak, C., and Gallo, B. *Critical Care Nursing: A Holistic Approach,* 6th ed. Philadelphia: J.B. Lippincott Co., 1994.

Medication Administration and I.V. Therapy Manual, 2nd ed. Springhouse, Pa.: Springhouse Corp., 1993.

Nursing97 Drug Handbook. Springhouse, Pa.: Springhouse Corp., 1997.

Skidmore-Roth, L. *Mosby's 1996 Nursing Drug Reference.* St. Louis: Mosby-Year Book, Inc., 1996.

Smetzer, S., and Bare, B. *Brunner and Suddarth's Textbook of Medical-Surgical Nursing,* 8th ed. Philadelphia: J.B. Lippincott Co., 1996.

Williams, B., and Baer, C. *Essentials of Clinical Pharmacology in Nursing,* 2nd ed. Springhouse, Pa.: Springhouse Corp., 1994.

Wong, D. *Whaley & Wong's Nursing Care of Infants and Children,* 5th ed. St. Louis: Mosby-Year Book, Inc., 1995.

Index

---

i refers to an illustration; t refers to a table; **bold** indicates pretest, practice, or review problem answers.

i refers to an illustration; t refers to a table; **bold** indicates pretest, practice, or review problem answers.